1001 little ways to spend less and look beautiful

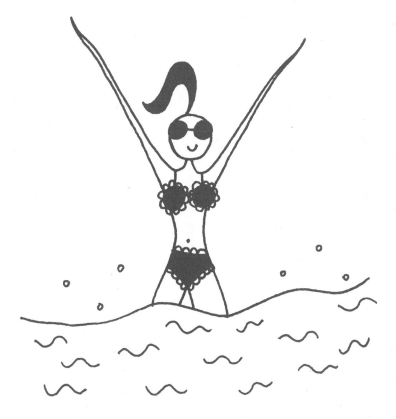

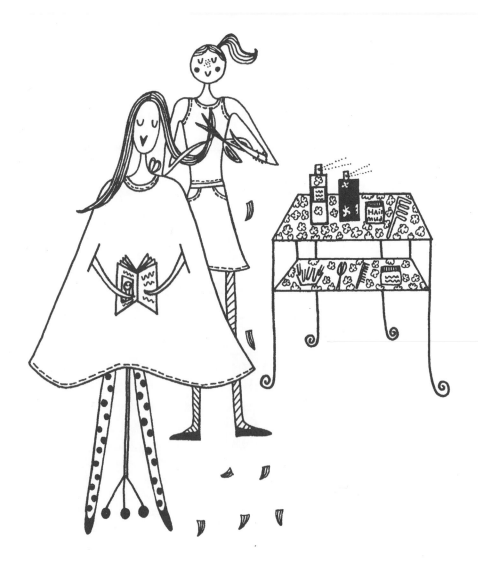

1001 little ways to
spend less and look beautiful

Caroline Jones

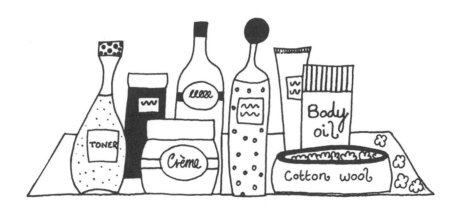

CARLTON
BOOKS

THIS IS A CARLTON BOOK

Text, illustrations and design
copyright © Carlton Books Limited 2009

This edition published by
Carlton Books Limited
20 Mortimer Street
London W1T 3JW

10 9 8 7 6 5 4 3 2 1

A CIP catalogue record for this book is available
from the British Library.

ISBN 978 1 84732 387 3

Printed and bound in Dubai

Senior Executive Editor: Lisa Dyer
Managing Art Director: Lucy Coley
Designer: Anna Pow
Copy Editors: Clare Hubbard and Nicky Gyopari
Production: Kate Pimm

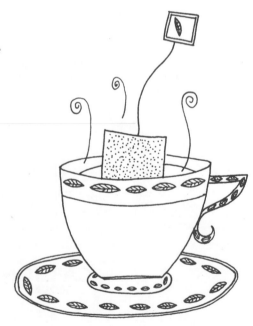

CONTENTS

introduction **6**

beauty basics **8**

cosmetics **42**

skincare **69**

haircare **92**

body beautiful **118**

therapies & treatments **152**

secrets & savings **198**

index **222**

INTRODUCTION

Would you like to discover the inside track on the beauty products that really work so you never waste money again? Or find out how to make your own indulgent skincare creams for a fraction of the cost?

From the gadgets and products worth spending on and those to avoid, to clever ways to blag great freebies and DIY spa treatments, this fabulous book contains 1001 amazing little ways to ensure you look a million dollars – without breaking the bank. It's also packed with advice on multipurpose make-up, getting better deals at the salon and secret celebrity money-saving tricks that will guarantee you always look beautifully groomed – whatever your budget.

Top ten little ways to spend less & look beautiful

34
ALL CREDIT TO THE CRUNCH
(see Mouth & Teeth Treats, page 15)

98
PAINT-STORE PARADISE
(see Beauty Tools, page 30)

169
LITTLE WHITE LIE
(see Budget Bridal Beauty, page 47)

185
A DYNAMIC DUO
(see Multipurpose
Products, page 50)

307
STRAWBERRY SCRUB
(see Skincare, page 76)

475
TANGLE-FREE TRESSES
(see Haircare, page 110)

548
SIMPLE SUGARING
(see Hair-Removal Hints,
page 125)

724
CHOCOLATE BLISS
(see Therapies &
Treatments, page 164)

796
CLEVER CAMOUFLAGE
(see Fake a Boob Job, page 181)

992
SAVVY SAMPLES
(see Final Freebies,
page 203)

grooming dos & don'ts

1 DO WEAR A HAT

Ultraviolet (UV) rays will dry out your hair, make it frizzy and cause split ends and breakage. Protect it by covering it up with a pretty hat in the summer months and save yourself loads of money on conditioning and frizz-fighting products.

2 DO CHECK YOUR POSTURE

Forget a fancy haircut or new designer dress – standing up straight with your shoulders back and your stomach pulled in is a free and instant beauty trick. You'll look more confident, taller and thinner.

3 DON'T LEAVE TELLTALE LINES

Regardless of how pricey your foundation is, nothing cheapens your look more than obvious tidemarks. Blending is the key, so keep a soft wedge-shaped sponge handy for around the jaw and hairline.

4 DO KEEP NAILS NEAT

You don't need to spend lots of money on a weekly manicure for pretty hands. Just make sure they're moisturized and your nails are a neat oval shape. Instead of always applying polish, invest in a nail buffer for natural gloss. It costs next to nothing and lasts for years.

5 DO TAKE GOOD CARE OF SKIN

A good skincare routine will help ensure you're consistently fresh-faced and gorgeous. There's no need to buy lots of expensive products – no-frills ranges from your local grocery or department store are actually less likely to unbalance your skin's delicate pH levels.

6 DO REMEMBER TO SMILE

When shown a range of different faces, studies show that people consistently pick out the smiling faces as being the most attractive – regardless of wrinkles, bad hair or other supposed defects. So practise your smile – it's a free and instant way to look more attractive.

7 DO PERFECT YOUR PLUCKING

There's no need to pay to have your eyebrows shaped professionally every time. Once you have the shape you want, simply check your eyebrows for new growth every few days and pluck any strays. Your eyebrows frame your face, which means that if they're in good shape you'll instantly look more groomed.

8 DO FIND YOUR MAKE-UP MUST-HAVE

You don't need to cover your face with a multitude of expensive cosmetics to look great every day. If your complexion is clear, all you need to do is brush on a coat of mascara and a touch of lip gloss for an instant groomed look. Save bright eyeshadows, blushers and lipsticks for special occasions.

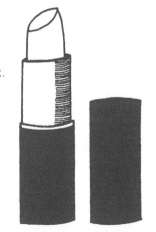

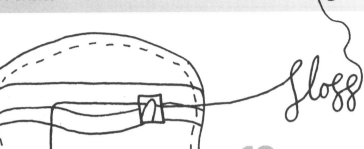

10 DO SPEND TIME, NOT MONEY

If you get up half an hour earlier, or start getting ready for a night out sooner, you'll have enough time to blow-dry and style your own hair – and save yourself a fortune on visits to the salon. If you need to learn how to get a professional blow-dry, ask your stylist for a lesson – it could save you a lot of money over the course of the year.

11 DO GUZZLE THE CLEAR STUFF

Drink as much water as you can throughout the day, especially during the winter months when you are less likely to be thirsty but central heating can leave you dehydrated. Drinking at least 2 litres (2¼ US pints) a day will not only ensure that your skin is hydrated and radiant, but it will also help to keep your eyes bright, your hair shiny and your lips moist.

9 DO LOVE YOUR TEETH

A great set of teeth will always make you look like a million dollars. And remember, prevention is always cheaper – so instead of spending money on whitening treatments, take good care of your teeth with thorough brushing and daily flossing.

12 DON'T RELY ON LIP BALM

Many people find that lip balm is an addictive habit and the more they use one the more they need it to keep lips soft and flake-free. Instead of constantly buying more lip balm, simply apply your normal facial moisturizer to your lips – it will soften them for longer and won't slide off. Make sure it doesn't get into your mouth and don't lick your lips!

13 DON'T GO OUT WITHOUT SUNSCREEN

We all know the sun damages the skin, yet we're all guilty of being lazy from time to time when it comes to applying an SPF before leaving the house. These days many moisturizers and foundations contain an SPF, so there really is no excuse. Just think of all the money you'll save on anti-ageing products.

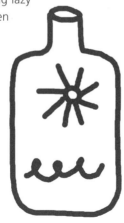

14 DON'T BE SEEN WITH CHIPS

It doesn't matter how smartly you're dressed or how perfect your hair is, chipped nail polish just screams of sloppiness. If you don't have time to redo the polish or don't want to spend money on a manicure, then remove all the old polish from your nails. Natural nails will look more groomed.

15 DON'T IGNORE SPLIT ENDS

Split ends instantly make your hair look a mess. Unfortunately, the only way to get rid of them is to cut them off. You can do this yourself by twisting your hair into small strands and snipping off the offending splits that stick out. Alternatively, an early trim costs a lot less than the drastic restyle you'll need if you let those ends get worse.

16 DON'T SLEEP IN MAKE-UP

Sleeping in your make-up is the ultimate beauty no-no. You'll end up having to spend loads on products to save your damaged, pimply skin. Keep a pack of face wipes by your bed for nights when you're just too tired to cleanse.

17 DON'T SQUEEZE

It can be hard to stop yourself, but the best way to tackle spots (pimples) is to dab them with antiseptic and then leave them alone. After all, it's harder and more expensive to hide a scar than a spot. Picking also pushes dirt deeper into your skin, resulting in prolonged redness.

18 DON'T FAKE IT TILL YOU EXFOLIATE

There's no need to spend on a salon spray tan – you can achieve the same results at home as long as you spend a little time preparing your skin. Always exfoliate and slather on loads of moisturizer otherwise your tan will look blotchy and uneven. Pay particular attention to your knees, heels and elbows and wear gloves to avoid orange palms.

19 DON'T FORGET YOUR FEET

Your feet may spend the winter hibernating in socks but if you continue to take good care of them, moisturizing regularly and trimming toenails, you won't need to splash out on a pedicure the next time you want to slip into a strappy sandal.

anti-ageing eats

20 GET BETA-SKIN

Nibbling on carrot sticks is an amazing way to fight wrinkles. Carrots are a cheap source of beta-carotene, an antioxidant that helps with the production of new, healthy skin cells and the shedding of old ones. Plus, beta-carotene fights free radicals, which damage skin and lead to premature ageing.

21 EAT A RAINBOW

Brightly coloured fruit and vegetables not only cost less than unhealthy snacks and ready meals, they're also rich in antioxidants, which ensure that nutrients and oxygen get to your skin cells to help prevent sagging, dull skin and protect against early wrinkling. Don't overcook veg, and eat them raw as much as possible.

22 FRUIT GOODNESS

Citrus fruits are a cost-effective way to get your daily dose of vitamin C, which helps produce collagen – the building block that keeps skin supple and elastic. Vitamin C also regulates the oil-secreting sebaceous glands to keep skin from becoming dry, strengthens capillaries to avoid spider veins and reduces the formation of age spots.

23 COMBAT CROW'S-FEET WITH CHICKEN

Chicken and turkey are great sources of high-quality, low-fat protein, which helps to keep your skin elastic and toned without breaking the bank. Try to eat the meat two or three times a week.

24 GET A FISH FACELIFT

Salmon is rich in omega-3 fatty acids, which help decrease inflammation and improve blood circulation, to help keep skin young, supple and radiant. Its natural oils also aid in the prevention of dry skin. Canned salmon saves precious money and is just as healthy as the fresh stuff.

25 DOSE UP ON DARK GREENS

Inexpensive dark, leafy greens such as bok choi, kale and spinach contain antioxidants called carotenoids that can help keep your skin looking youthful by helping to block sun damage – a key cause of wrinkles.

26 GRAPE EXPECTATIONS

Red wine contains the powerful anti-ageing antioxidant resveratrol, which helps maintain a youthful-looking complexion by fighting damaging free radicals. Cabernet Sauvignon grapes have the highest concentration of antioxidants. However, sticking to one glass a day makes the bottle last longer and prevents excess alcohol from drying out the skin.

27 GO NUTS

Almonds pack more goodness than many more expensive pills. They contain selenium, vitamin E and other essential fatty acids to help keep your skin supple and hydrated. Vitamin E also assists in the regeneration of skin cells to reduce the signs of ageing.

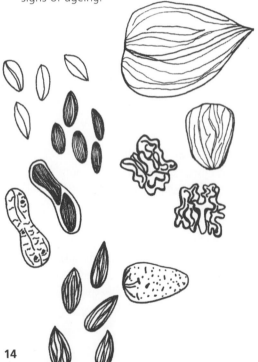

28 CHOCS AWAY

Dark chocolate is one of the richest sources of skin-boosting antioxidants, and eating it is actually a more efficient way to absorb them than applying an overpriced cream. Choose a variety with at least 70 per cent cocoa solids for the best results. Try dipping fresh fruit in melted dark chocolate for the ultimate wrinkle-fighting dessert.

29 SKIN-PROTECTING SELENIUM

Brazil nuts are rich in selenium, a trace mineral that helps keep the skin safe from the sun and also encourages skin elasticity. Buy a big bag and then eat just three or four a day to provide you with the recommended daily amount.

30 TONING TOMATOES

This shopping staple contains more lycopene, one of the most powerful anti-ageing antioxidants, than any other food. Lycopene can be more readily absorbed when the tomatoes are processed, so tuck into soups and pasta with tomato sauce for a simple and cheap skin-boosting lunch.

31 IRON OUT CREASES

It's estimated that only one in ten women get enough iron in their diet. An iron deficiency can leave you feeling tired and looking pale with dry, itchy skin. Top up your stores by tucking into lean red meat and seafood. For a budget veggie alternative, you can find iron in spinach, lentils and fortified breakfast cereals.

32 ANTI-AGEING GARLIC

This pungent bulb costs very little but is an effective tool in combating wrinkles and encouraging skin healing. The beneficial anti-ageing properties of garlic are at their strongest when the garlic is raw, but if you want to cook it, leave it out for ten minutes after chopping before frying. This ensures the garlic retains more of its important compounds during the cooking process.

mouth & teeth treats

33 TEETH LOVE TEA

Tea contains polyphenols, which fight plaque-causing dental bacteria and ward off cavities, and makes it harder for bacteria to cling to your teeth. Green tea contains the highest amounts, but you'll still get plenty from a cheap cup of standard tea.

34 ALL CREDIT TO THE CRUNCH

The credit crunch might be causing you headaches but crunchy foods such as fresh apples and celery naturally remove red wine, tea or coffee stains from the enamel of your teeth – at a fraction of the price of expensive stain-removing toothpastes.

35 A ROOT SOLUTION

Radishes contain fluorine – a trace element that strengthens tooth enamel. Try them sliced in salads and stir-fries.

36 AN APPLE A DAY KEEPS...

This inexpensive snack increases saliva
secretion, which protects your teeth against
cavities and decay. A post-dinner apple
makes for an instant 'brush', but never
actually brush your teeth straight after
eating fruit as the combination of scrubbing
and fruit acid can wear away tooth enamel.

37 MILKY GOODNESS

To protect your teeth from decay eat plenty
of low-fat live yogurt. This budget snack is
high in calcium, which helps to keep your
teeth cavity-free and is a natural bacteria
fighter. Research also shows that people
who get enough calcium in their diet are
less likely to develop severe gum disease.

38 A CHEESY GRIN

Make a small slice of hard cheese part of
your diet every other day. Cheese helps to
stop bacteria from growing in the mouth
and prevents cavities. Be careful not to
overdo the amount as cheese is high in
unhealthy saturated fats!

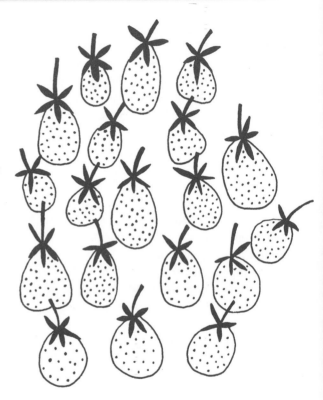

39 STAIN-REMOVING STRAWBERRY

These clever berries have a natural
bleaching effect on your teeth. Simply
wipe over teeth for a sparkling smile.

skin-savers

40 WHEATGERM WIPEOUT

To wipe out spots (pimples) include 2–3 tablespoons of wheatgerm in your diet each day. It is sold by the bag for next to nothing in health stores and is rich in skin-clearing B vitamins and vitamin E. Sprinkle on to cereal, yogurt or cottage cheese.

41 GET AN E-SAVER

Vitamin E-rich creams, such as those containing hazelnuts, almonds, avocado and sunflower seeds, are better for your skin than many more expensive creams. Not only do they help prevent dry skin, they will help protect it from sun damage and aid the repair and reduction of scars and stretch marks.

42 DARK CIRCLE-FIGHTING DUO

Forget pricey eye creams – a combination of vitamin C and iron will help reduce dark circles under your eyes. Combine lean beef with red, yellow and orange peppers in a tasty stir-fry for your double dose.

43 BERRY GOOD NEWS

Looking a little pale? Berries such as cranberries and blueberries are rich sources of bioflavonoids – natural antioxidants that strengthen the cells that make up the blood vessel walls. This increases blood circulation, giving you a beautiful, healthy glow without recourse to expensive fake tan.

44 GOOD SKIN ON TAP

You might get bored with being told this, but because the skin is 70 per cent water, keeping it properly hydrated is vital if you want it to look good. And these days, it's better for the environment and your bank balance to get your eight glasses a day from the tap (faucet). Add a splash of fruit juice or cordial to liven up the flavour.

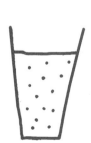

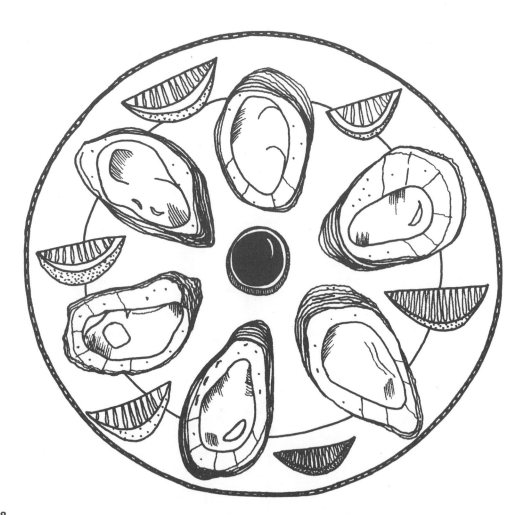

45 SEAFOOD FIGHTER

Zinc is a potent infection fighter that can help tackle acne. People who suffer from spots (pimples) often have low levels of zinc, so tuck into seafood to top yours up. If seafood seems expensive you can swap oysters for eggs, which are also high in zinc.

46 DITCH THE DAIRY

Some studies link full-fat milk to an increase in spots (pimples). Non-organic milk is another suspected culprit. Try switching to organic skimmed milk for smoothies, cereals and tea. Your blemish-free complexion is worth the extra money for the slightly more expensive milk, and think how much you'll save on skin treatments in the long run!

47 KITCHEN CURE

Apple cider vinegar is concentrated with enzymes that help you shed dead skin cells, leaving the skin soft and supple. Dilute with an equal amount of mineral water and use as a cut-price revitalizing toner (start with a 5:1 ratio to see how your skin reacts to it).

48 BROCCOLI BOOSTER

This super-veg has as many nutrients as lots of expensive multivitamins. Broccoli is a good source of vitamin A, which helps reduce oil production; vitamin K, which reduces the formation of bruises; and vitamin C, which is a powerful antioxidant that prevents fine lines and wrinkles.

49 SCAR SOLUTION

Beauty products designed to aid healing are very expensive. Eating plenty of vitamin C-rich fruit can help scars heal more quickly. Good sources include citrus fruits such as lemon, orange and grapefruit, but the richest source is kiwi fruit. Just one kiwi fruit has twice the vitamin C content of an orange.

50 GET GORGEOUS WITH GREEN TEA

A fraction of the price of a fancy skin cream, green tea is loaded with vitamins, minerals and antioxidants. This makes it effective in fighting inflammation and premature ageing. Drink three to four cups a day.

hot hair

51 HEALTHY HYDRATION

Drinking water is a great free tonic for your locks as it encourages healthy hair growth and keeps the follicles nourished and flexible.

52 BEANS FOR A BEAUTIFUL BOB

Some experts believe that an overload of toxins in the body leads to dull hair. So flush out your system on the cheap by eating plenty of fibre-rich foods such as lentils, beans and wholegrain cereals.

53 SILKY SILICA

Silica is a mineral that is important for keeping your hair elastic, shiny and healthy. It can be found in oats, cucumber skin, onions and bean sprouts, which means a healthy and economical diet of porridge (oatmeal) for breakfast and salad for lunch.

54 DITCH THE DIET

Not only can faddy diets cost a fortune in groceries, cutting out major food groups such as dairy or carbs can starve your body of vital nutrients and disrupt hair growth.

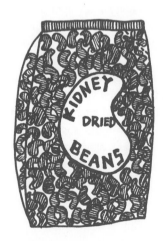
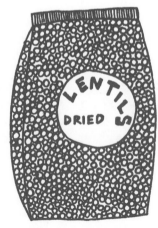
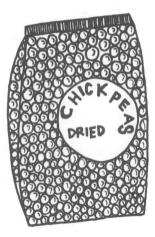

55 MINERAL MAGIC

Not getting enough zinc in your diet can hinder the body's formation of the hair protein keratin, damaging your hair follicles. Feed your hair by eating more zinc-rich foods, particularly shellfish, fish and cereals.

56 GO GREEN FOR GLOSS

Forget salon hair conditioners – save cash by gorging on green vegetables. They're rich in B vitamins that promote the secretion of a natural hair conditioner called sebum from the hair follicle which leads to super-shiny hair. Other sources of vitamin B are eggs, milk and poultry.

57 THE POWER OF PROTEIN

Protein is vital for healthy hair growth and prevents breaking and splitting. Eating fish ensures the necessary protein intake for a magnificent mane, while also providing shine-enhancing omega-3. Nuts are an even cheaper dose of omega-3.

nails

58 DURABLE DAIRY

A daily intake of calcium is important for strong nails, so by eating plenty of yogurt and other low-fat dairy products you can soon stop spending money on stick-ons.

59 PROTEIN POLISH

Keep nails strong and moisturized by eating plenty of protein. Protein helps in the production of keratin – the substance our nails are made of. Skinless chicken breast and lean turkey are healthy sources while tuna and beans are an even cheaper option.

60 BOOST WITH BIOTIN

Biotin is another building block for healthy nails. So dump the expensive perfect-nail pills and tuck into biotin-rich foods like eggs, soya and cauliflower. A diet rich in biotin is guaranteed to help strengthen and thicken your nails.

61 PUMP IT UP

If you notice that your nails are brittle, or have developed vertical ridges, your body may be suffering from lower than optimum iron intake. Snack on pumpkin seeds for a quick and cheap iron boost.

62 TOUGHEN YOUR NAIL TIPS

Eating turkey is a better way to make your nails more robust than any strengthening nail polish you can buy. This lean meat is rich in selenium, which is vital for growing strong, healthy nails.

63 NAIL BOOST

Fresh carrot juice is rich in vitamin A, calcium, phosphorus and B vitamins – all of which help strengthen nails. And think how cheap a bag of carrots is!

64 ZAP WHITE SPOTS WITH ZINC

A lack of zinc – not calcium as many people think – is the cause of white spots on your nails. Fish and seafood are the richest sources of zinc, but if you're not a fish lover, pine nuts and pecans are good too.

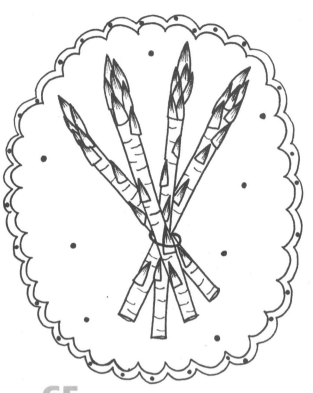

65 STRENGTHENING SULPHUR

Asparagus is rich in sulphur, a mineral that's vital for strong nails as it strengthens the nail bed. Other sources include seafood, onion, garlic and cabbage.

66 BRILLIANT B12

Insufficient intake of vitamin B12 can lead to nails that break easily and are distorted in shape. Liver and eggs are great sources of this beauty-boosting nutrient.

67 POPEYE POWER

There's no point spending money on manicures if your nails are weak and brittle. Spinach is rich in essential B vitamins, which are important for helping nails to grow stronger. Eat raw in salads or lightly steamed.

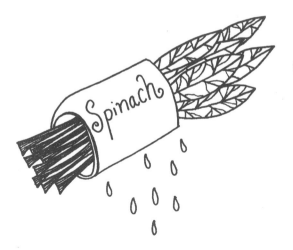

budget shopping

68 DISCOVER WHAT'S IMPORTANT TO YOU

Make two lists – one detailing the products you really can't live without and one of the items that you don't use very much or really don't need to use. For example, if you have dry skin you'll need a good moisturizer but can quite happily go without toner. Or if you hate your pale lashes, you'll need mascara but perhaps wouldn't miss lipliner. You may end up halving your beauty bill.

69 LOYALTY IS NOT ALWAYS A VIRTUE

Just because you can't live without your favourite expensive moisturizer, it doesn't necessarily mean you have to buy all your skincare products from the same range. Rather than being fiercely loyal to one brand, experiment with supermarket own-brand products for basic beauty items such as deodorant, toner and eye make-up remover.

70 PRIORITIZE THE PROBLEM

Is your hair dry or greasy? If it's dry it might be worth buying a budget shampoo and spending a bit more on conditioner. However, if your hair is greasy it makes more sense to go for a shampoo that targets your problem and to save money on a budget conditioner.

71 NEED NOT WANT

Learn to prioritize. Yes, that metallic eyeliner is tempting but it's not going to make you look any prettier if you haven't got a good canvas on which to apply it. When money is tight, make sure you have the basics to keep you groomed and glowing before splashing out on sparkly extras.

72 SOMETIMES IT PAYS...

Many department stores and supermarkets offer reward cards on which you collect points for every purchase you make. Collect points while buying essentials like soap and toothpaste and when you've collected enough you can use them to get a free beauty treat.

73 BULK-BUY

Take advantage of promotions. Stock up on six months' worth of shampoo and conditioner the next time your favourite line of products is on offer at a reduced price. However, some products – mascara, for example – have a short shelf life so don't buy them in bulk or they'll go to waste.

74 CUT BACK ON NEUTRALS

It's worth splashing out on expensive brands when buying brighter eye and lip shades as cheaper make-up sinks into your skin more, making the colour less vibrant on application. But when buying neutral colours, don't splash the cash – you'll get the same effect from cheaper ranges.

75 SIGN UP FOR SAVINGS

Many make-up brands offer regular benefits, such as free full-size samples, to people on their mailing lists. If you don't want spam clogging up your inbox, open a new email account specifically for mailing lists – and log on whenever you're in need of a freebie!

76 SUPERSIZE SHAMPOO

When buying shampoo or face wash, you may save money in the short term by buying smaller bottles, but it's often wiser to go for the biggest available size if it's a product you already know and trust. Try working out the cost wash for wash to discover how much you'll save.

77 KEEP IT SIMPLE

Trying every product in the quest for a perfect complexion may be tempting, but overdoing the experimental purchases is one of the biggest – and priciest – beauty mistakes. Keep it simple with a good and trusted cleanser, moisturizer and sunscreen – the rest is unnecessary.

78 DON'T GET KITTED OUT

Make-up brands are always trying to create complete product packages that look like a bargain, but don't get sucked in. Chances are you'll only end up using two or three things from the kit, and you could have saved money and got more of the things you really liked by buying them individually.

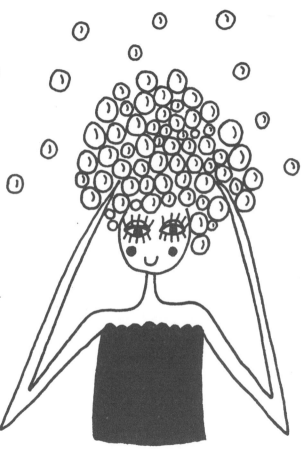

79 PARE DOWN

There's an alarming
array of mascaras
out there – ones that
lengthen, volumize,
curl or separate. Don't
be tempted to buy one
of each. You'll only
use one at a time.
Also, once opened
mascaras must be
used within three
months, so having
unused options is
simply wasteful.

80 COMPARE THE MARKET

If you have seen the perfect shade of eyeshadow or lipstick at an expensive make-up counter, ask for a sample and then compare it to cheaper brands. Chances are you'll find exactly the same colour for a fraction of the price.

81 SAVE ON SHAMPOO

It's essentially just soap, so expensive miracle formulas are unlikely to give you noticeably better results than a basic version. Most supermarkets and chemists do their own-branded ranges these days with products targeted specifically for different hair types, which are just as good.

82 COMPARE INGREDIENTS

You love your expensive moisturizer because it leaves your skin super-smooth, but are you sure you're paying for a quality product and not just for packaging and the name? Compare the ingredients with cheaper brands and you're sure to find a cheaper product that works just as well.

83 SMOOTH MOVE

There's no point splashing out on an expensive body moisturizer, as you want to be able to slather it on daily without worrying about how much you are using. Inexpensive body lotions and oils will do just as much to moisturize your skin as the cheaper brands – but they just might not smell as expensive!

84 BE BRAND SAVVY

If you are looking for a particular brand of make-up, don't just buy it from the first place you see it. Different stores sell the same products at different prices, so shop around. And don't forget the internet – specialist beauty-product websites and eBay offer massive savings.

85 DON'T GET SUCKERED

Special offers such as 'two-for-one' are only bargains if you're actually going to use the products. If you're just going to put them in the back of a drawer and forget about them that's not saving!

86 BUY COLOUR IN BULK

If you know you want to achieve a certain look – say smoky eyes – it can actually be cheaper to buy an eyeshadow palette that contains all the shades you'll need to create the look rather than individual colours.

87 GET GLOSSY FOR LESS

You're either going to lick lip gloss off, or leave it behind on coffee cups or people's cheeks, whether it's expensive or cheap. Save your pennies and buy a budget one!

88 CHEAPER FOUNDATION

You don't need an exact colour match for tinted moisturizers, or even much in the way of coverage, so save your money and buy a cheaper high street version for results that are just as good.

89 DON'T BE A MAGPIE

Are you a sucker for pretty packaging? Well, the truth is cheap doesn't have to mean ugly. You can keep your bathroom looking beautiful by transferring cheap products into pretty bottles.

90 NAIL IT DOWN

The more expensive nail varnishes often contain stronger colour pigments so you can apply fewer coats and the colour won't chip as quickly, which means a small bottle will go a long way. They are also more likely to glide on smoothly for a better finish.

91 A NATURAL BLUSH

In bronzes and blushers, the powder tends to be of a finer grade in more expensive brands, so the colour will look more natural on your cheeks and should last longer. Cheaper brands are more likely to clump and streak.

92 CONCEAL THE TRUTH

Cheaper brands of concealer tend to dry out quickly, which can make the blemish you were trying to conceal stand out even more, or accentuate those undereye bags.

93 SPEND ON SELF-TANNERS

It's worth spending a little more to avoid the nasty smell of cheaper brands and ensure a streak-free finish – you'll still be spending less than if you had it applied professionally.

94 KEEP KOHL

Even expensive eyeliner can smudge, and the ingredients in the cheaper versions are almost identical if you compare them.

95 SPEND FOR YOUR AGE

Younger skins can get away with cheaper foundation, but if you're hoping to hide wrinkles and age spots it's worth paying more as the higher-end formulations tend to be more hydrating and contain the latest light-reflecting technology.

96 ANY KIND WILL DO

Cosmetic powder doesn't have to be expensive – the translucent version of any budget brand will do the trick. Luxury brands may be ground finer and available in various shades, but a translucent variety covers most people's needs.

97 TREAT YOUR FACE

A good day facial moisturizer will leave your face smooth and therefore cut down on the amount of foundation you need as well as any primer products you may have to buy.

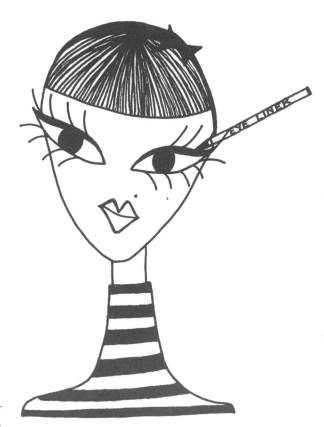

basic beauty tools

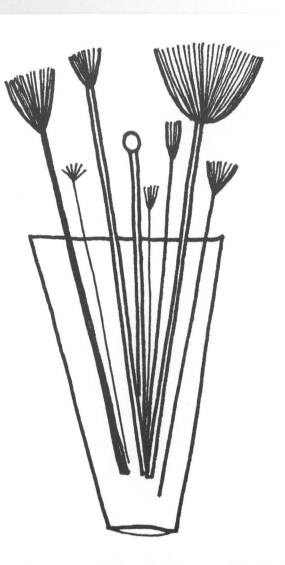

98 PAINT-STORE PARADISE

If you go to an art supply store you'll be able to find brushes in the same shapes and sizes as make-up brushes but for half the price. Be careful though – not all paintbrushes are suitable for use on your face so make sure you choose brushes with soft bristles and choose natural fibres rather than synthetics.

99 BEAUTY IN A BOX

Store all your make-up in an airtight container to seal out moisture, which can change the appearance and texture of some make-up. Excess moisture can even lead to make-up going off, meaning you will have to throw it away and replace it.

100 WASH AND BRUSH UP

The key to long-lasting make-up brushes that don't need constant replacing is regular cleaning. Soak your brushes in hot water with a mild liquid soap, then rinse under cold running water. Leave out on a paper towel to air-dry. Snip away frayed ends to ensure flawless application.

101 BALLS IN A BAG

We tend to throw away make-up bags when they inevitably get grubby but you can ensure your make-up bag lasts longer simply by putting two or three cotton balls in it. The cotton balls attract all of the loose powder or lipstick in your bag, keeping it cleaner for longer.

102 CLEVER COTTON

Cotton buds (swabs) are inexpensive but invaluable as they make a very versatile make-up tool. They are great for applying eyeshadow, blending in foundation and concealer and for fixing eyeliner and mascara mistakes; you can also use them for touching up manicures.

beauty gadgets: not worth your cash

103 BODY-TONING PADS

If you want to lose weight these gadgets just won't help. Even if their mild toning effect does anything in the way of tightening, because fat sits on top of muscle you won't see any difference unless you diet and exercise too.

104 HOME-TANNING SYSTEMS

You can achieve just as good results with the latest spray tan product bought from a pharmacy – aerosol sprays are best on hard-to-reach areas.

105 ELECTRIC MANICURE SET

Electric nail files are pricey and can actually split your nails. It's much easier and cheaper to do it manually, with the ever-reliable emery board under your own steam.

106. HEATED EYELASH CURLERS

Just blast your normal eyelash curlers under your hairdryer for a second instead. But to avoid singed eyelashes make sure the curlers are not too hot before using them.

107. FACIAL SAUNA

You can achieve exactly the same results with a bowl of warm water and a towel over your head. Add a few drops of essential oil to the water and you can create your own soothing facial sauna for a fraction of the price.

108. HOT STYLE

Blow drying wet hair and then styling it can cause damage and lead to breakages. It's much better to let your hair dry naturally before using heated stylers.

109. FEET TREATS

Foot spas are waste of cash with weakly powered bubbles! Simply fill a plastic bowl with enough warm water to cover your feet and add some softening bubble bath for an equivalent experience.

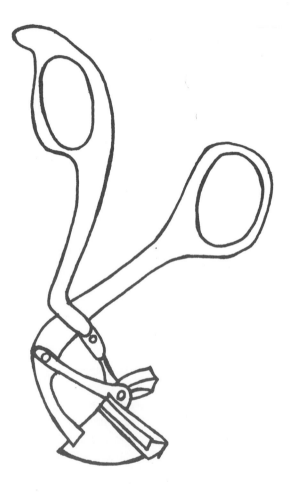

110 MASSAGE GADGETS

When it comes to massages, nothing beats the human touch. Skin-on-skin contact adds to the relaxation factor and you can achieve a greater range of pressure and strokes with your hands than with any fancy, costly gadgets.

111 ILLUMINATED COSMETIC MIRROR

Beauty mirrors can be expensive and bulbs need replacing. It's much better to apply make-up in natural light anyway, or you can risk looking like a clown when you leave the house. To get an even better effect than an illuminated cosmetic mirror, simply position your mirror next to a window and place a lamp nearby.

112 INDUSTRIAL-STRENGTH HAIRDRYER

Hairstylists use expensive super-strength hairdryers with powerful motors because they blow-dry so many clients every day, but you don't need that much power to achieve the same finish at home, and these types can damage hair if used regularly.

beauty gadgets: worth every penny

113 HAIRSTYLING SCISSORS

You can't use any old scissors to trim your fringe (bangs). Cutting fabric and paper blunts the blades so they'll snag and split your hair. A pair of professional-quality blades will save you a fortune in salon trims.

114 MAGNIFYING MIRRORS

They make everything – from plucking your eyebrows to applying your make-up – so much easier. So investing in a good magnifying mirror will make it simple to take care of your beauty at home.

115 ELECTRIC TOOTHBRUSH

Nothing says 'well groomed' better than a pearly white smile. An electric toothbrush shifts much more bacteria than brushing with a regular brush, saving you a small fortune in dentist bills.

116 PEDOMETER

Clipped onto your belt this gadget will count the amount of steps you do a day. Think of it as your own motivational personal trainer – but much cheaper! Aim to do 10,000 steps a day to stay in shape.

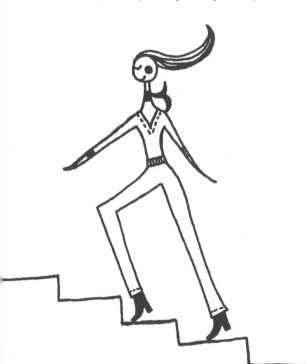

117 HAIRDRYER WITH SETTINGS

Having different heat settings will set your style and protect your hair from excessive heat exposure. Look out for hairdryers with ionic conditioning to help reduce frizz and static. Just think how much money you'll save on salon blow-dries.

118 HAIR-REMOVAL SYSTEMS

These home systems are perfect for small areas of the body. Needle-free, they use gentle laser or pulsed light and although they're not cheap to buy, in comparison to having regular electrolysis at a salon you'll save a fortune.

118 EXERCISE DVDS

If you want a cheap aerobic workout, exercise DVDs are great. You'll be able to afford a huge variety for less than one month's gym membership and class fees. Or make it even cheaper and sign up to a DVD rental website.

active ingredients worth every penny

120 BIKINI TRIMMER

Specifically designed for use on sensitive skin, this gadget allows you to trim and shape with precision. Investing in one of these nifty gadgets will save you a fortune each month on salon bikini waxes.

121 CERAMIC STRAIGHTENERS

Worth the money, ceramic straighteners protect hair from static and snagging. Plus, they heat up quickly, removing the need to go over the same section of hair numerous times, therefore they are gentler on your hair. Also, by wrapping your hair around the straightening iron you can create bouncy curls. Two tools for the price of one!

122 DECENT TWEEZERS

A good-quality pair of tweezers will last you forever. You'll be able to shape perfectly arched eyebrows without the help of a professional, so these inexpensive tools will pay for themselves in no time.

123 CERAMIDES

A natural substance within the skin, ceramides reduce natural water loss of the skin by forming a protective barrier and also help to hold the skin's cells together in a firm, smooth structure. Ceramides can also be produced synthetically and added to skincare products, and have been used in products since the early 1990s. They have proven anti-ageing benefits.

124 RETINOIDS

These vitamin-A derivatives are one of the few ingredients shown to combat the serious signs of ageing. They penetrate skin more deeply, to strengthen and replenish collagen and elastin, plump up skin and unclog pores.

125 DIHYDROXYACETONE

Present in self-tanners, this carbohydrate reacts with amino acids found in the top layers of the skin to create a shade of brown within two to six hours, and can build colour depth with every reapplication. It has a long history of safe use. A cost-effective and healthy way to tan.

126 ALPHA-LIPOIC ACID

A powerful antioxidant and anti-inflammatory that occurs naturally in your cells and helps reduce under-eye puffiness. An excellent ingredient to look out for in eye creams.

127 VITAMIN E

This nutrient plays a crucial role in protecting skin cells from environmental damage on an everyday basis, but it is also excellent for calming stressed, sun-damaged skin.

128 ALPHA-HYDROXY ACIDS (AHAS)

AHAs, originally derived from fruits, reduce fine lines, smooth skin and remove blemishes. They also help exfoliate without the need for scrubbing. AHAs need time to work – go for products that you leave on the skin, such as moisturizers and masks. They can be harsh though, so avoid them if you have sensitive skin.

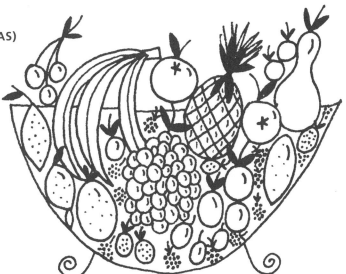

129 ZINC OXIDE

Zinc oxide is a proven UV blocker. It's the basis of many sunscreens and is particularly good if you have sensitive skin.

130 BETA HYDROXY ACID (BHA OR SALICYLIC ACID)

Found naturally in plants, this is a great ingredient for blemish-prone skin. It has antibacterial properties and gently exfoliates deep inside your pores to prevent outbreaks.

131 CAFFEINE

Caffeine helps ingredients penetrate the skin and can stimulate the circulation. It's most widely used in cellulite treatments, but is also useful in gels to combat puffy eyes.

132 VITAMIN B3

Also known as niacin, B3 has been shown to prevent skin from losing water, keeping it hydrated. Worth paying for.

ingredients that might be worth paying for

133 HYALURONIC ACID

This plumping agent is found naturally in the skin and helps it retain water and stay moisturized. If you have dry skin it could be worth paying for products that contain it.

134 COENZYME Q10

This nutrient is found naturally in the body and is thought to strengthen cells. In theory, applying it should help protect against wrinkles caused by free radical damage, but few studies so far back this claim.

135 ELASTIN

This is the stuff that gives skin youthful flexibility. However, adding it to cosmetics has never been shown to affect the elastin in skin or to have any other benefit. Don't pay lots for this addition.

136 VITAMIN C

When applied to your skin vitamin C is said to fight wrinkle-causing free radicals. However, effectiveness varies greatly from person to person, so before splashing out on a vitamin C skincare product it's a good idea to try a sample.

137 ANTIOXIDANTS

Although they have anti-ageing properties when eaten in food, currently there's no proof that antioxidants in skincare products actually benefit the skin. Check how much your product actually contains as companies often put only tiny amounts in their formulas.

138 COLLAGEN

Collagen naturally works with elastin to give skin its youthful, plump appearance, but this appearance can deteriorate with sun damage and ageing. However, while applying it to your skin synthetically in a face cream will attract moisture to your skin, there's little evidence that it will stimulate your skin's production of collagen.

139 PANTHENOL (VITAMIN B5)

This ingredient is used in hair products to attract moisture to your hair and smooth the surface, making it more light reflective, resulting in shiny locks. Worth checking for, but don't pay over the odds.

140 MINERAL OIL

This is one of the best-known moisturizers and one that hardly ever causes allergies. However, it's incredibly cheap to produce so don't pay a lot for a cream that has mineral oil as the main ingredient.

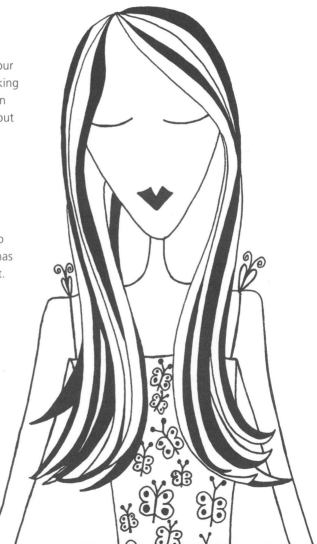

ingredients that are a waste of money

141 HUMECTANTS

These moisturizing additives are actually more important in preventing your product from drying out than for keeping your skin moisturized!

142 ENZYMES

Used in skincare for exfoliation and to inhibit free-radical damage. However, enzymes are picky about what conditions they will work in and often need other enzymes, called coenzymes, to function, or a specific temperature or pH. Unlikely to do much, so save your cash.

143 OXYGEN

Oxygen boosts skin cell turnover when you breathe it in, not when you apply it to your skin. Steer clear!

144 ALL NATURAL

When a product claims that it contains only natural ingredients, it's not saying that the contents are safer for your skin. All it really means is that the ingredients were not produced chemically. However, this doesn't mean that it will be better for your skin or never cause allergic reactions.

145 PEPTIDES

These flash-sounding ingredients haven't been proven to fight ageing, so it's not worth paying more for them.

146 POLYPHENOLS

Again, these are great antioxidants with anti-inflammatory benefits when consumed in things such as green tea, but they've not yet been shown to offer the same benefit when slathered on your skin.

147 DNA

Including the building blocks of all life in a skincare product is pointless because as an ingredient it can't affect a cell at a genetic level – and nor would you want it to!

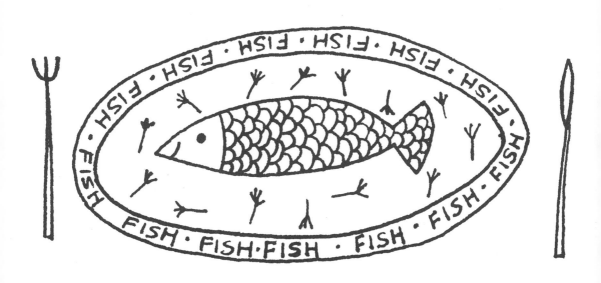

148 OMEGAS-3 AND -6

Essential fatty acids such as omega-3 and 6 give you
glowing skin when eaten in oily fish and nuts, but
they haven't been shown to have a significant effect
when applied to your skin's surface.

make-up makeover

149 END OF LINES

Ask your local beauty salon for end-of-line lipsticks and nail polishes. They'll often offer them at a discount to clear the shelves for new stock.

150 DITCH THE FANCY PRODUCTS

Let's face it, tried-and-tested products may not be fashionable but they've been around for years, they don't break the bank and they work. And that's why they've been around for years.

151 ONLINE MAKEOVER

A whole host of beauty websites now offer a free online tool (often called a Virtual Makeover) that lets you see how you would look with different hairstyles, lipstick colours, sunglasses, hats etc. You simply scan in a picture of yourself and experiment to your heart's content. It's free and fun.

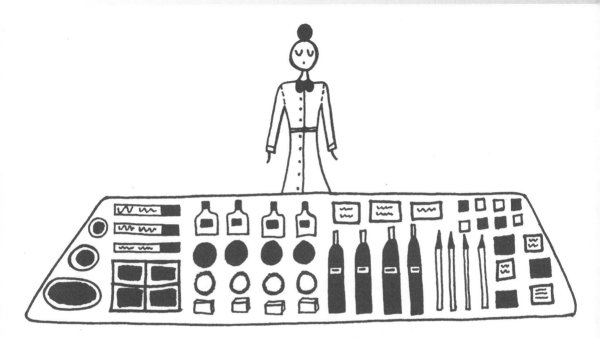

152 COUNT ON COUNTERS

Department store make-up counters are always happy to offer free makeovers so why not make the most of them by booking one just before a special occasion? Don't feel you have to buy anything, but you will sometimes get a discount on any purchases that you make.

153 COLOUR ME CUT-PRICE

Makeover salons that help you decide on colours for clothes and make-up are often much quieter in the late summer months and early winter (Christmas, New Year and spring tend to be busiest). Look for special offers or simply drive a hard bargain and demand a discount – starting at half price.

154 COLOUR-MATCH YOURSELF

If you can't afford to visit a special salon to be told which colours suit you, buy a book of colour swatches. By holding the colours up against your face you get a great idea of which shades of eye make-up, lipstick and blusher to experiment with.

155 MAKEOVER MATES

We all have make-up mistakes, freebies from magazines and unwanted presents lurking somewhere, but don't throw something away just because the colour doesn't suit you – it might be perfect for a friend. Have a product swap party and invite friends to bring their make-up mistakes along. When inviting them make it clear that the make-up must be new and unsealed. Sharing make-up or using old make-up that may have deteriorated can be a health hazard.

156 DON'T ASK, DON'T GET

When splashing out your cash on a new exfoliator, see if the girls behind the make-up counter will throw in a complimentary moisturizer for you to use afterwards. They can only say no!

157 BE A GUINEA PIG

Offer yourself as a test dummy at your local beauty college. Trainee make-up artists can practise creating a look on you for free. Chances are you'll look fabulous, but don't worry if it all goes horribly wrong – it will easily wash off!

158 WRITE A LETTER

It's always worth writing in to newspapers and magazines for a reader makeover. They often have to find at least one real-life case study for every issue and so welcome volunteers. You'll be pampered and preened (and photographed!) for free.

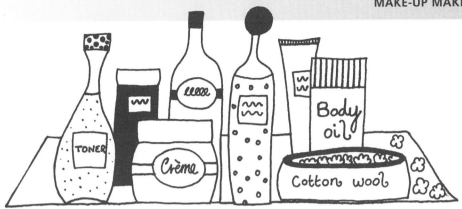

159 THROW A MAKE-UP PARTY

Companies selling make-up door-to-door will often organize make-up parties and come to your home if you can guarantee a certain number of guests. So invite the girls, open a bottle of wine and make it an evening. Anything you buy will be discounted.

160 UNEARTH YOUR ANTIQUES

Every woman's got one – a huge drawer that holds lots of unused make-up. Now's a great time to tip it all out. You'll be amazed by how much you own; how much is usable; and how much you actually like. Mascara and eyeliner should only be kept three to six months, so these need to go if older than this.

161 MAKE YOUR OWN WAVES

No need to have a perm in a salon to get a curly new look. Instead, do it at home by splitting hair into sections and wrapping each section around a rag. Pin up until dry or leave overnight and you will wake up to beautiful, tousled tresses.

162 CHANGE ONE THING

People assume you need to change your whole make-up bag for a new look, but just tweaking one small thing can have an amazing effect – and save you money. Investing in one new staple, such as a green eyeliner or a different shade of lipstick, will refresh your other products.

163 SAVVY SAMPLES

It's important to see foundation in natural light to ensure you've chosen the right shade. Ask for samples at beauty counters to give a new colour a trial run. This will avoid a costly mistake and you may well end up with enough for a few nights out!

164 BENEFITS OF A RESTYLE

If you can't afford to splash out on a full cut, a cheap and effective way to restyle is to have your fringe (bangs) cut. A fringe is nearly always in fashion and can really change your look, plus hairstylists charge a fraction of the price of a whole haircut to create one.

budget bridal beauty

165 STICK TO WHO YOU KNOW

Going to your usual hairstylist can save you money, especially if you're particularly friendly, as the chances are he or she might offer it as a wedding present!

166 DOUBLE UP

Get your hair and make-up done together by someone who offers both as a package. You can often halve your costs this way – and the stylist will think about creating a whole look for you with hair and make-up working together.

167 A GROUP CURE

Make an appointment to get manicures and pedicures done together with your bridesmaids. Let the salon know you are a bridal party – you can often negotiate a group discount or get the bride's treatments free.

168 LET YOUR HAIR DOWN

Why is that women who always wear their hair down get pushed into having an expensive 'updo' on the day that doesn't really suit them? If you love your hair loose, wear it that way and pay for a simple blow-dry at half the cost.

169 LITTLE WHITE LIE

Don't always be quick to say you're getting married. Companies often immediately quote you their 'bridal' price, which can involve adding extra zeroes. This tactic is especially useful if you're not having a big white wedding – you could just be celebrating a special birthday.

170 CHECK THE HOTEL

If you're having your ceremony or reception at a hotel, check out their spa bridal packages as they will often offer them to you at a discount if you're getting married there. This way you could get all your beauty needs – nails, hair and make-up – done on site for less.

171 PHONE A FRIEND?

Do you have a friend whose make-up always looks just-left-the-salon standard? Why not ask them to do your make-up on your wedding day?

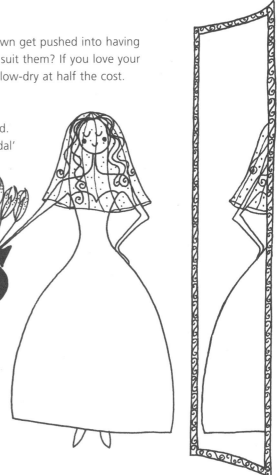

172 DO-IT-YOURSELF

Brides often feel pressured to have their make-up done professionally on the day, but you could save yourself a heap of money by practising now so you can master how to do it yourself. Spend a couple hours every weekend in the lead-up to the wedding experimenting with different looks until you achieve one you like. This will also avoid that over-made-up look that so many brides regret when they look back at their wedding photographs!

173 AVOID HOME VISITS

You can save money just by going to the beauty salon or hairstylist yourself on the morning of your wedding rather than having them come to you – a service they always charge more for.

174 ASK YOUR MATES

Ask all your friends who've got married recently for recommendations. Then treat it as you would a pricey home-improvement job – get three quotes and pick the one you feel most comfortable with.

multipurpose products

175 LINE THEM UP

Want a smoky-eyed look without buying a new eyeliner? With your eye closed, touch the tip of a mascara wand along the lash line of your upper eyelid, then quickly smudge the dots with a cotton bud (swab) for smoky definition.

176 SUPER STAINS

Many make-up brands now offer multipurpose stains that can be applied to both the cheeks and lips. This saves the cost of buying two products and creates a more natural rosy glow.

177 MULTIPURPOSE MASCARA

Get more out of your mascara by using it to groom and define eyebrows as well as lashes. Go for a clear mascara or pick a natural-looking colour, as black may be too harsh for some complexions.

178 THRIFTY THREE-IN-ONES

NARS invented the original multipurpose colour stick, which can be used on lips, cheeks and eyes. Now other ranges, including supermarket own brands, have jumped on the three-in-one band-wagon, so you can get this make-up must-have for a fraction of the cost.

179 HANDY HIGHLIGHTERS

Highlighters are a great budget buy as they can be used in so many ways. To lift your eyes – apply along the brow bone; for a wide-eyed look – apply to the inner corner of your eyes; for a healthy glow – blend along your cheekbones; and for full lips – blend along your Cupid's bow.

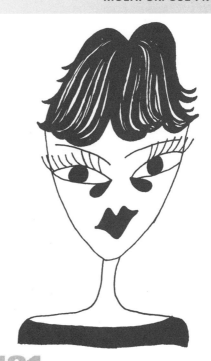

180 EXOTIC EYELINER

Eyeshadow is available in a far wider selection of colours than eyeliner. Be creative and save money by turning your favourite shade of eyeshadow into an eyeliner. Simply dampen an eyeliner brush with water, dip it into the shadow and run along your lashes.

181 PERFECT HIDEAWAY

Don't despair if you've run out of concealer, try the ring of foundation that collects around the neck of your foundation bottle. Moisture that was in the foundation will have evaporated, so the remnants are more concentrated and will offer better coverage – just like concealer.

182 CHEEKY EYES

Warm tones really open up the eye area.
So instead of buying a new eyeshadow,
apply powder blusher in a soft bronze,
peach or rose colour to your eyelids up to
your brow bone. Using the same colour on
your eyes and cheeks will even out your skin
tone and give you a natural-looking glow.

183 LUSCIOUS LIPS

Don't want to waste money on yet
another lipstick? Cream or powder blusher
can be dabbed on lips with a finger to
create a soft, sensual look. For a creamier
texture, top the blusher with clear gloss or
petroleum jelly.

184 LIPPY CHEEKS

Lipstick can also be used as a blusher –
but bear in mind that lipstick contains far
more pigment than blusher. To avoid going
overboard, start with a tiny dab, then
gradually build up the colour. Blend well
with your fingertips or a cotton bud.

185 A DYNAMIC DUO

For the ultimate budget-friendly look,
make up your whole face using only
bronzing powder and petroleum jelly. Use
the bronzer as blusher and eyeshadow,
then mix it with some petroleum jelly
for a golden lip gloss. Finally, slick some
petroleum jelly on your lashes and brows
for shine and definition.

186 NOT JUST FOR BABIES

There's a host of overpriced fancy body
oils and sprays on the market, but all you
really need is a little baby oil. Rub
it in after a
shower or add
a few drops
to your bath
water for
super-soft
skin. It
also works
as cuticle
cream.

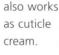

187 WISE WIPES

Keep on hand a packet of three-in-one face wipes that cleanse, tone and moisturize, or at least cleanse and tone. By choosing a multipurpose product rather than three separate ones you'll save money and time.

188 MULTIPURPOSE PETROLEUM JELLY

Petroleum jelly is the original multipurpose product. Use it as lip balm or to tame wild brows. Or run some along your collarbone for a sexy shimmer. Petroleum jelly can also be used as a moisturizer or to tame frizzy hair – just remember a little goes a long way and you don't want to look like an oil slick!

189 SUPER-STRAIGHT

Forget lots of fancy hair tools – you can achieve a multitude of styles with just a thin straightening iron. As well as poker-straight locks you can create corkscrew curls by wrapping your hair around one plate of the iron, working your way up towards the roots. You can also vary the look depending on how tightly you wind your hair or by brushing out the curls to create soft waves.

190 WONDER POWDER

Bicarbonate of soda (baking soda) dries up spots (pimples) and makes for a great gentle facial exfoliator when mixed with a little warm water. Gently massage the paste into your skin for 10–15 seconds, then rinse off and pat your face dry with a clean towel. Bicarbonate of soda also relaxes your muscles when sprinkled into hot bath water. You can even rub it on to your teeth for a natural way to a whiter smile.

191 TALENTED TEA TREE

Tea tree oil is naturally antibacterial, anti-fungal and antiseptic – and cheap. As well as drying up spots (pimples), this clever oil soothes and speeds up the healing time of cold sores and a few drops added to your shampoo will help get rid of dandruff.

192 MAGIC ANTI-STATIC SPRAY

Hairspray can be used to tame unruly clothes as well as unruly hair. The aerosol spray can prevent static build-up, so when wearing a silky dress simply spritz a bit of hairspray on to your tights (pantyhose).

193 MELLOW YELLOW

Lemons are a fabulous fruit. Soak nails in a bowl of warm water and lemon juice to whiten them, or use this mixture to remove fake tan stains. Lemon juice is also excellent for bringing out highlights – spritz on to hair, leave to dry for half and hour, before going out in the sun for 2–3 hours.

194 REPURPOSE PRODUCTS

If you run out of essential items some products can double up – bronzer can be used as blusher or eyeshadow and mild shampoo as a make-up brush cleaner.

195 SAY ALOE!

Keep a pot of soothing aloe vera gel handy. It costs very little from the health food store and can be used for calming brows after plucking, soothing sunburn and reducing puffy eyes (check the product you have bought is safe to use around eyes). Plus, rub it into your scalp after conditioning and leave for 15 minutes and it will help thicken fine hair.

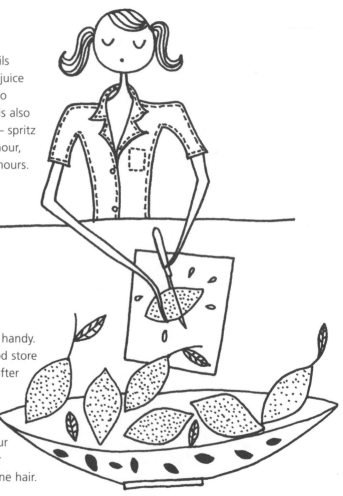

196 HANDY FRIZZ FIGHTER

Hand lotion doesn't just soothe dry mitts, it can also smooth dry hair. Apply the lotion to hands as normal and then simply run your hands over the frizzy area. The moisturizers in the lotion will instantly smooth out frizz, leaving behind a glossy sheen.

197 WELL POLISHED

Always keep a bottle of clear nail polish in your handbag (purse). Not only does it add smart gloss to nails in seconds when you've no time for colour, it will also stop runs in tights (panty hose) from getting worse if you dab a little on to the ends of the run.

198 A POINTED RESPONSE

Invest in a medium-sized brush with a slanted tip for the ultimate multiple-use tool. You can use the angled edge for eyeshadow and the fatter side for blusher and loose power. Do be sure to clean your brushes regularly and between different uses.

bases & concealers

199 CLEVER COMBO

Why pay for a separate foundation and moisturizer, when you can get one product that does both jobs: a tinted moisturizer? To ensure a natural look, test it down the centre of your nose to make sure it settles well around your pores.

200 LIQUID GOLD

To get to the last bit of liquid concealer in a tube with a wand applicator, use a concealer brush or a clean lip brush.

201 SHADES OF SUMMER

Instead of buying a new foundation in the summer months when your skin is a darker shade, mix your old one with a little bronzer and moisturizer in the palm of your hand and apply to give skin a healthy glow.

202 FINGERTIP FOUNDATION

There's no need to splash out on special sponges for foundation application. With practice you can achieve a flawless finish using only your fingers. Fingers can reach places that sponges can't and it's also easier to avoid getting foundation in your eyebrows and hairline.

203 COLOUR CODED

A cheap foundation will work just as well as an expensive one if you choose the right shade. Don't bother testing it on the back of your hand – the skin colour is too different. Instead, pop a blob onto your jawline. Provided it blends seamlessly into your neck, it's the right choice regardless of price.

204 THE UNDERTONES

Rather than slapping on lots of beige concealer, go for a small dab of a shade with an undertone that will neutralize your blemish or dark circles, and will last a lot longer. A green undertone counteracts redness, yellow conceals dark circles and lilac lifts sallow skin.

205 FATTEN UP YOUR FOUNDATION

To make your foundation last longer, mix a small amount with your daily moisturizer before applying. You'll achieve the perfect tint of colour that spreads on easily to even out your complexion.

206 GET TO THE BOTTOM OF THINGS

If you can't get to that last bit of foundation or squeeze the last liquid make-up out of the tube, place it under hot running water for a few seconds. The warmth should help it slide out.

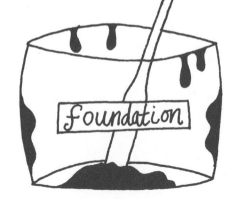

207 BACK TO LIFE

Has your foundation become caked and dry? Pour a few drops of alcohol-free toner into your foundation bottle and shake. It will last that bit longer and you'll be toning your face at the same time.

208 DON'T CAKE IT ON

If your skin's in pretty good condition there's no need to cover your whole face with foundation. Just apply concealer where you need it to hide dark circles or blemishes. As the old saying goes 'less is more'.

209 STICK TO IT

Get the last bit of concealer stick out of the bottom of the tube with a toothpick – but make sure you apply it to your hand first. Don't use the toothpick on your face!

210 AU NATURALE

If you're not going out of the house, skip the make-up. There's no need for a face full of cosmetics if you're going to be cleaning or relaxing. Not only will this save on make-up, it will give your pores a break from clogging.

211 LIGHTEN UP

We all love YSL's Touche Éclat for hiding our dark under-eye circles but it's not cheap. Check out other ranges, including supermarket own-brand cosmetics, as nearly all of them do an imitation. Not as expensively packaged perhaps, but many are just as effective.

212 DITCH THE EXTRAS

Some cosmetic companies charge as much for a face primer as for their foundation – promising that it will ensure a smooth application and long-lasting finish. Don't be fooled – your normal moisturizer will do exactly the same job.

213 BLEMISH SOLUTION

If you suffer from oily skin and blemishes, think twice before buying overpriced medicated foundations. Stick to the one you love and simply add a few drops of witch hazel. Known for its astringent properties and for tightening pores, it's often used in toners for oily skin and is available in pharmacies.

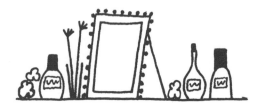

powders

214 BE SIZE SAVVY

When you shop for foundations and concealers, don't just compare the prices. Write down how many millilitres/ounces they give you and figure out the cost per millilitre/ounce to accurately compare prices. If you don't do this the prices – and bottle sizes – can be deceiving.

215 DON'T HIGHLIGHT PROBLEMS

Again, there's a myth that foundation needs to go all over the face. It doesn't. Foundation can be spot-applied to the areas where you need to even out your skin tone, such as grey under-eye bags or blotchy cheeks. This gives a more natural look to your make-up and means you use less.

216 SKIP A STAGE

If you have dry or mature skin don't bother with face powder. Foundation doesn't need 'setting' these days to stay put and powder can settle in creases and dry areas to give an unflattering effect.

217 DOUBLE-DUTY BEAUTY

The latest mineral powders are made from natural ingredients, are gentle on skin, and replace the need for foundation as they offer great matt coverage. Perfect for oilier skins.

218 TREATMENT MAKE-UP

Buy powder that contains an SPF and moisturizing ingredients so you get more bang for your buck.

219 MAKE USE OF LEFTOVERS

Once you've finished your loose or pressed powder, the sponge applicator makes a great oil blotter for greasy hair roots between washes.

220 PUT A CAP ON IT

Some make-up companies recommend buying loose power to keep at home and a pressed powder compact to keep in your handbag (purse). Save money by just buying the far more versatile loose variety and a retractable brush that can hold a little powder in the cap.

221 POWDER RUN DRY?

Loose powder tends to be more expensive than pressed powder but if you don't wear much, you can make your own. Mix baby powder with one part powder from a cheap powder compact. Choose the compact powder in a colour darker than your skin and mix to get the right shade.

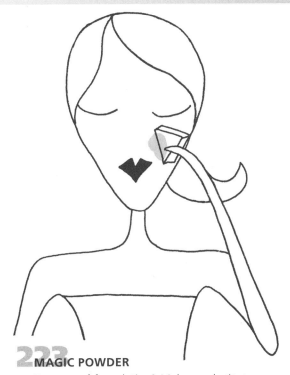

222 BE A PEARLY QUEEN

To make a 'luminescent' face powder for evenings, add a little white or peach frosted eyeshadow to a small amount of face powder in your palm and apply with a brush. If you prefer, you can just dust your face very lightly with any of these frosted powders using a brush.

223 MAGIC POWDER

Run out of foundation? Make a substitute of two parts face powder to one part unscented hand lotion. Mix only enough for a single use in the palm of your hand. It has a nice finish, but the oil in the lotion can darken the colour, so you may need to add some baby powder to lighten it.

224 ADD SOME DEPTH

If you have old loose power that's a shade too light so it's not getting used, add some bronzer or blusher to it. Just add a little at a time and mix to create a bespoke colour that is perfect for your skin tone.

225 CLEVER CONTAINERS

Wash out pretty powder pots once they're empty and use them to store earrings or cotton balls.

eyes

226 AFTERNOON CLEAN-UP

A cotton bud (swab) dipped in petroleum jelly or lip balm is a great way to clean up smudged eye make-up, thereby avoiding that bad mid-afternoon habit of washing everything off and reapplying – a sure-fire way to use up products twice as fast. Make sure you don't get any in your eyes!

227 TAPE FOR PERFECTION

Low-tack masking tape can safely create the perfect lines for precise liquid eyeliner. The trick is to cut a piece about 2.5 cm (1 in) long and peel it off the skin of your hand once or twice to lose a little of the stickiness. Then place at the desired angle on the corners of your eyes.

228 GOOD FOUNDATIONS

You don't need to spend extortionate amounts on expensive bases and primers that promise to stop your eyeshadow creasing and flaking. Simply apply your foundation to your eyelid as a base to keep your shadow in place all day.

229 GO FOR GOLD

Gold shimmer eyeshadow can be used as a highlight all over the face. Run it along the bony bit just below the eyebrow or dab it down the centre line of the nose and at the top of the cheekbones. But try to stick to only two areas of shine at a time!

230 MAKE WAVES WITHOUT CURLERS

You don't need expensive eyelash curlers to curl your lashes. Just bend your lashes back from the root with your finger, and hold them there for a few seconds. Set the curl with a coat of mascara.

231 DON'T PUMP IT UP

Do you pump your mascara wand in and out of the tube every time you apply it? Well stop it now! Not only does this overload the brush and lead to clumpy lashes, it also forces air into the tube causing the mascara to dry out more quickly.

232 SHADOW FIXES

Keep your eyeliner in place, and reduce the need for constant reapplication, by patting dabs of black eyeshadow on top of it. This will stop your eyeliner smudging or bleeding and will keep your precious kohl stick lasting that bit longer.

233 WIPE AWAY MISTAKES

Forget expensive eye make-up removing wipes, which can often sting and irritate the face. Low-cost baby wipes, which are often used by make-up artists, work just as well and are often a lot gentler.

234 REFRIGERATOR FRESH

Try keeping eye pencils, lipsticks and nail polishes in the refrigerator. This will stop them drying out and make them easier to apply. It should also prevent the tips of pencils and lipsticks from breaking off.

235 RETURN BAD ADVICE

If you buy a product on the advice of a counter assistant and then find it's not suitable or doesn't do what was promised, it's much easier to get a refund than buying 'off the rack' in a pharmacy.

236 EYE DYE DO-IT-YOURSELF

Instead of going to a beautician, tint your eyelashes and eyebrows with a home kit that is far cheaper than a trip to a salon.

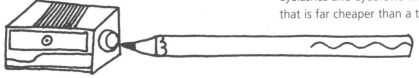

237 REFRESH MASCARA

You can refresh dried-out mascara by heating with a hairdryer for a few seconds. However, make sure you change your mascara every three to six months to avoid nasty eye infections.

238 BUDGET MASCARA

Of all the make-up products, mascara is the one you can scrimp on because the secret to good mascara is the brush not the formula. Many cheaper brands have very good mascaras.

239 DON'T LASH OUT

Fond of false lashes? Be economical and get a better effect by snipping the lashes in half and placing them only on the outside of the eye. Don't place them at the very end of the lash line, though, or your falsies are liable to droop – leave a 2 mm (1/16 in) gap instead.

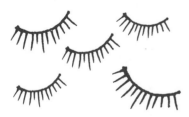

cheeks

240 FIND YOUR PERFECT PARTNER

Don't waste money on lots of different shades of blusher – if you find the right shade to complement your skin tone you can wear it day and night. Fair-skinned ladies should go for pink and tawny tones, redheads will glow in peach and coral shades, and olive skin tones suit brown and copper shades.

241 TOTAL TAN

Wear a bronzer all year round. We tend to think of it as a summertime treat but it's a Hollywood secret that keeps many an ageing starlet from looking her age. And the subtle, healthy glow will save you lots of money on tanning treatments.

242 TONE IT DOWN

Powder blusher too bright? Don't throw it out. Crush it up and mix in a little brown blusher, matt brown eyeshadow or matt powdered bronzer.

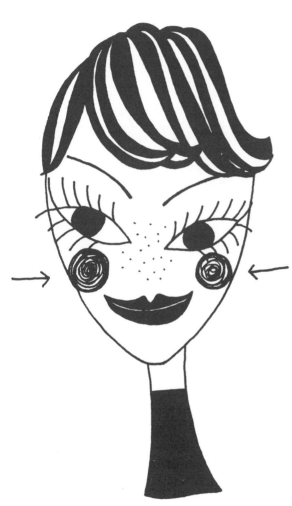

243 FIRST FLUSH

Don't overdo it with the blusher – you only need to use a tiny amount provided you apply it correctly. The area to apply it to is the 'apples' of your cheeks, where you blush, funnily enough!

244 LIGHTEN UP

Powder blusher too dark? You can lighten it a couple of shades by crushing it up and mixing in a little baby or face powder.

245 HAVE A REFILL

Many make-up companies now make eco-friendly, reusable compacts with refills that can cost a lot less than buying a new compact every time.

246 DO A REPAIR JOB

Eyeshadow, blusher or powder that comes inside a compact may start to break up and fall out in time. This can be fixed by adding a little surgical spirit (rubbing alcohol) and smoothing the powder back in place with a butter knife. Let the powder dry completely before using.

lips

247 GET LIPPY

There's no need to pay extra for long-lasting lipstick. Even the cheapest lipstick can last all night if you apply it well. Use a lip pencil all over the lips, then apply face powder to set the pencil. Top with a coat of lipstick, then blot your lips by pressing them together on some tissue before applying a second coat.

248 DON'T BE FLAKY

Instead of splashing cash on a lip primer, use a touch of petroleum jelly before applying lipstick. Dip an old toothbrush in petroleum jelly and gently rub it over your lips in a circular motion to scrub away all the flaky bits.

249 TEA TONER

Tea can help your lips retain moisture and appear smoother. Simply press a used teabag to clean lips, while it's still warm, and use to clean for five minutes.

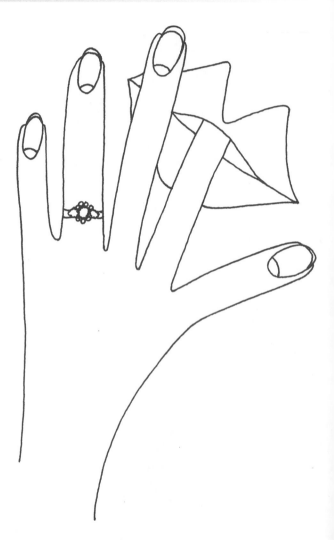

250 LINE BY LINE

A lipliner can be used in the place of lipstick to colour in the entire lip. As well as taking up less space in your handbag (purse), the colour lasts longer.

251 LONG-LIFE LIPSTICK

Lipstick can last for up to two years, depending on the brand, so don't throw it out when you only have a little nub left. Scrape it into an empty, sterilized lip-gloss or eyeshadow pot instead. If you're feeling creative, you could even mix different shades to make your own colour. Apply with a lipbrush.

252 SHIMMER AND SHINE

Make your own sparkly lip gloss: stir 1 heaped teaspoon of petroleum jelly, ¼ teaspoon of hot, boiled water and 1 teaspoon of sugar together until the sugar is dissolved. Then add some pink or red food colouring and a pinch of edible glitter. Let the mixture cool then scoop it into an empty lip-gloss container. Use within one month.

253 MIX IT UP

You can make your own lip gloss from the end of a lipstick. Put a little petroleum jelly and a little of your leftover lipstick in an empty, sterilized lip-gloss pot. If it doesn't blend together well, put it in a microwave-safe container and heat for a few seconds.

254 KEEP IT CLEAN

When applying a clear gloss over coloured lipstick, always apply using a cotton bud (swab), not the applicator in the gloss tube. Dip the cotton bud (swab) just once into the gloss and then apply to your lips. This prevents the rest of your gloss becoming discoloured and you having to throw it away before it's finished.

255 SPICY LIP PLUMPER

Cinnamon encourages blood flow, and is the key ingredient in many expensive lip plumpers. Blend a drop of cinnamon oil with a tablespoon of olive or almond oil and rub it onto your lips. It will make your lips tingle and give them a natural fullness.

256 BETTER BRUSH STROKES

Use a lip brush to apply your lipstick. With a lip brush, you will apply a thinner layer of lipstick than if you were to apply it straight out of the tube. Plus you can scrape out every last bit of your lipstick with your lip brush, preventing leftovers. Waste not, want not.

257 THE PERFECT SHADE

Have a too-bright lipstick you'd like to salvage? Apply a medium-brown lipstick or lipliner pencil over the top to tone it down.

258 NATURAL OILS

A little olive oil will soothe dry, chapped lips as well as any store-bought balm. Simply dab it on with your finger.

259 CAP IT

Taking care of your lipsticks will make them last longer. To avoid squashing it, make sure your lipstick is rolled all the way down before putting the cap on. Also, make sure the top clicks into place to keep out air and reduce the growth of bacteria.

260 BROWN SUGAR

If your lips are dry, a budget, soothing balm can be made by mixing a little brown sugar with honey. The sugar will gently exfoliate dead skin cells while the honey is great for rehydrating dry skin.

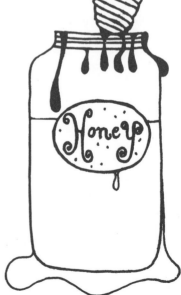

261 GO GREEN

If you recycle your old lipstick tubes some companies, such as MAC, will give you a new lipstick for free (if you return six empties).

262 LIP SERVICE

If a broken lipstick is too mangled or misshapen to go back in the tube smoothly, use a small knife to transfer the lipstick to a plastic art palette. You can pick up artists' palettes at your local art store for next to nothing.

brows

263 ASK A FRIEND

Don't want to pay to have your brows plucked but scared of making a mistake? Get a tweezer-experienced friend who always has well-shaped eyebrows to help you the first time.

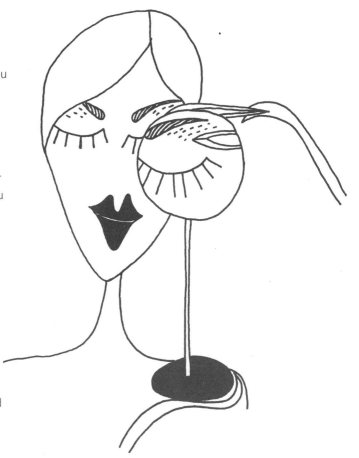

264 PROFESSIONAL SHAPING

Forget the brow bar and learn to shape your brows yourself. Here's a foolproof brow plan. Hold a pencil flat along the side of your nose; where it crosses your brow line is where your brow should start. Next, tilt the pencil so it forms a line from the corner of your nose past the outer corner of your eye. This is where it should end. Start plucking at the side nearest your nose and work outwards, removing a continuous line of hairs. Never pluck hairs from above your brow line.

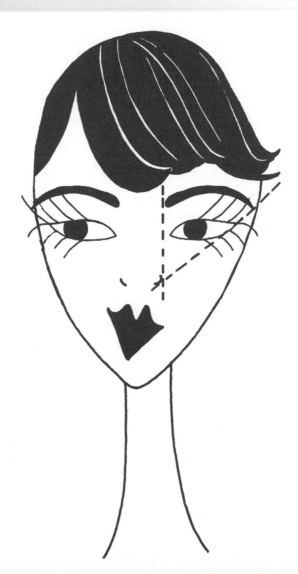

265 WISE WAXING

Home-waxing kits are relatively inexpensive, and do-it-yourself eyebrow waxing is easy once you've got the hang of it, plus it can last for weeks. Brush your eyebrows into place with a toothbrush, then apply wax in the same direction as the hair growth. Pull the skin taut and remove the wax against the direction of hair growth.

266 FAKE IT

If you have pale eyebrows, create the illusion of a strong brow with an eyebrow pencil rather than splashing out on semi-permanent make-up. To make it last the whole day simply use the eyebrow pencil first, then apply a matching powder shadow on top to set the colour.

267 GET TO THE POINT

Use an artist's knife with a fresh blade to carefully sharpen the point of eye pencils – it'll go that bit further to the bottom than if you use an eye-pencil sharpener.

268 BRING BLUNT TWEEZERS BACK TO LIFE

If your eyebrow tweezers are blunt, don't buy new ones – simply sharpen them by rubbing sandpaper along the edges.

269 ICE ICE BABY

You can buy special numbing creams, but a cheap way to prepare brows for plucking or waxing is to run an ice cube over them first.

270 DON'T FORGET YOUR TOOTHBRUSH!

You don't need to buy a special brush for your eyebrows or a product to hold them in place. Put a bit of hairspray or a dab of hairstyling gel on a recycled toothbrush and use this to tame your brows.

271 CHECK YOUR DRAWERS

There's no need to buy a special eyebrow pencil – chances are you already have an eyeliner or eyeshadow in the right shade that can be used to fill in brows. If you have a pencil that's too hard, warm the tip up by rubbing it between your fingers.

cleansing & care

272 CLEVER CLEANSING

If you cleanse your skin properly you'll save a load of money on blemish treatments and super-creams. Always wash your hands first – dirty palms make for clogged pores. Be especially gentle around your eyes, as dragging on this skin will lead to wrinkles and ageing crow's-feet.

273 GET CLARIFICATION

'Clarifying' mists and lotions often contain harsh ingredients such as acids and alcohol, which could make your skin feel sore and look blotchy. Cheaper products that don't make these claims may actually be better for your skin. Check the ingredients and make sure they're alcohol-free.

274 TONE UP

Most store-bought soaps are alkaline relative to the skin. A dirt-cheap way to redress this balance is by using diluted vinegar as a toner.

275 KITCHEN CLEANSER

Why buy an expensive cleanser when you can make one at home that's suitable for all skin types? This simple mixture will cleanse, tone and smooth: mix 1 teaspoon of honey with 1 teaspoon of natural (plain) yogurt. Apply to damp skin, wash gently and then rinse with warm water.

276 SIMPLE SOAP WILL DO

Don't waste money on expensive, fragranced soaps. Perfumed soap will only make dry skin worse and can often trigger allergies. Try a cheaper, unscented moisturizing soap instead.

277 FRESH MILK CLEANSER

Cucumber and milk are common active ingredients in many pricey cleansers. To make your own facial cleanser warm about 100 ml (½ US cup) of milk and add the juice of half a cucumber. Apply to the face using cotton balls. Gently sweep up the face until the skin feels clean and fresh. This is particularly good for dry or sensitive skins.

278 DEEP CLEAN

Make your daily cleanser last longer and work harder by turning it into a deep cleanser. Mix a dab of it with a pinch of oatmeal, then gently massage the mixture in circular motions on to your face. Rinse with warm water and pat dry.

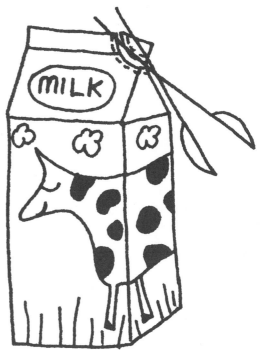

279 MILD MAKE-UP REMOVER

Common vegetable oils are great for removing non-waterproof eye make-up. Grapeseed oil is the least likely to cause irritation. Apply using soft cotton pads, then rinse thoroughly with warm water.

280 SOME LIKE IT COOL

If you shower or wash your face with water that is too hot it will damage the skin's natural moisture balance, so it becomes dry and in need of more moisturizer to keep it hydrated.

281 SPRINKLE SOME SALT

If you suffer from oily skin, then common table salt is a great way to reduce the oiliness. You can mix it with olive oil to make a cleanser or add a teaspoon to warm water to create a mild scrub.

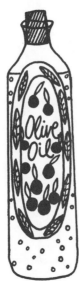

282 QUALITY NOT QUANTITY

A good cleansing routine should not need to be repeated more than once a day – doubling the life of your products. Cleanse at night and simply splash lukewarm water on to your face in the morning.

283 MILK IT

There are plenty of expensive oil-controlling lotions available, but not many actually work. But there's a matt miracle hiding in your medicine cabinet – milk of magnesia. Pour one or two drops onto a cotton ball and lightly pat all over your face to remove any hint of sheen.

284 BLOOMING MARVELLOUS

Store-bought toners often contain alcohol, which can dry the skin. Save money by making your own and you'll know exactly what you're applying. Boil 250 ml (1 US cup) of water and pour it over some rose petals. Leave for an hour with a lid on, then strain into a spray bottle. Lightly spritz on your face after cleansing. Store in the refrigerator for up to a month.

285 SAY NO TO LUXURY CLEANSERS

Rather than buying an overpriced cleanser, spend your money on quality products that actually spend time on your face, like a moisturizer. Remember, with a cleanser, you're just washing it down the sink.

286 STRAWBERRIES AND CREAM

For a cheap face-brightening mask: blend 50 g (⅓ US cup) of ripe strawberries with 470 ml (½ US pt) of milk and strain through a piece of muslin (cheesecloth). Using a cotton ball, smooth the liquid onto your face, leave for ten minutes, then wipe clean with a damp facecloth. The acids in the milk and the strawberries brighten dull skin.

287 PORE-TIGHTENING TOMS

Don't waste money on fancy pore-tightening treatments for blemished skin. Purée one unripe tomato and add 1 teaspoon of honey. Gently massage into your face, then rinse. The tomato acts like an astringent to tighten pores and remove excess oil, while the honey will soften the skin. Avoid using on sensitive skins.

288 LOOK BEYOND THE BOX

Don't be sucked in by fancy packaging or the wild scientific claims made in some ads. The key to a good cleanser or moisturizer is the active ingredient, not the label – most dermatologists will recommend products you can find in any supermarket or pharmacy.

289 DEWY NOT TAUT

Over-cleansing not only drains precious products, it can leave your skin feeling taut and can reduce the effectiveness of your skin as a natural barrier, leaving you vulnerable to problems that include rashes and acne. After light cleansing your skin should feel dewy rather than tight.

290 STIMULATE YOUR SKIN

Specialist brushes – including sonic brushes! – that stimulate your skin before cleansing are the latest fad, but you can replicate the effect of the bristles simply by rubbing your face with an ordinary facecloth. Wet the cloth first and gently make small circles to boost circulation.

281 DE-STRESS

Stress is terrible for your skin. According to the American Academy of Dermatology, it can trigger skin disorders such as acne, hives, eczema, rosacea, cold sores and psoriasis. It has also been shown to impair skin barrier function and dehydrate skin. Rather than treat the symptoms it's much more cost-effective to eliminate the cause, so find time to relax. Practising yoga poses, meditation and breathing, for example, has been shown to lower stress levels.

282 CAMOMILE CLEANSE

Soothing camomile is a good choice for sensitive or blotchy skin – and it costs the price of a tea bag! Dip one into warm water before gently massaging it in tiny circles around your face to reduce redness.

283 SKIP THE TONER

We all know the 'cleanse, tone, moisturize' mantra but if your budget is tight, consider skipping the middle step. Toners can actually dilute the good effects of a moisturizer. Use a splash of cold water instead.

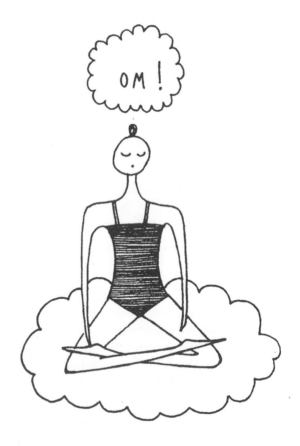

scrubs & exfoliators

294 SEEDS OF GOODNESS

Sunflower seeds, rich in vitamin E, make an excellent facial scrub. Mix 1 tablespoon of ground sunflower seeds with a few teaspoons of water to create a smooth paste. Massage gently into your skin and then rinse well.

295 EXFOLIATE EVERY TWO WEEKS

Save your favourite facial scrub and your skin by cutting down on your exfoliating routine. A gentle scrub every two weeks is enough for most skin types.

296 ORANGE APPEAL

Don't throw away your orange peel – let it dry, grate it and add 2 tablespoons to 1 tablespoon of oatmeal. Mix with cold water to create a paste, apply to your face, then gently rub off when dry, for a refreshing scrub.

297 REFRIGERATOR SKIN SCRUB

With a secret ingredient of alpha-hydroxy fruit acid, this homemade exfoliator removes dead skin cells to reveal soft skin. Mix 55 g (1/4 US cup) of sugar with two or three chopped tomatoes and 2 tablespoons of natural (plain) yogurt or sour cream. Gently massage onto your face, then rinse.

298 A SPOONFUL OF SUGAR...

Sugar scrubs have become increasingly popular, but why pay top dollar for them when you can make your own? Mix 1/2 teaspoon of sugar with a tiny bit of olive oil or honey. Lightly massage into your skin until the sugar melts away and finish by rinsing off thoroughly.

299 HONEY AND LEMON SOOTHER

Mix 1 tablespoon of honey, 2 tablespoons of finely ground almonds and 1/2 a teaspoon of lemon juice together and rub gently onto your face. Why? Well, the honey helps to moisturize, the almonds exfoliate and the lemon helps diminish redness and blotches. Rinse off and pat dry.

300 ADVOCATE AVOCADO

The next time you have avocado save the large stones (pits) and let them dry out for a few days. Grind them down to a powder using a coffee grinder to create a natural exfoliator that can be mixed with any cleanser for a deep clean.

301 SEA SALT SCRUB

A little sea salt sprinkled on a damp facecloth can make for a great exfoliator and pore unblocker, especially if you have greasy skin because salt naturally combats oiliness. Avoid, however, if you suffer from delicate or sensitive skin.

302 GET STONED

In the bath or shower, try rubbing a pumice stone over the pores on your nose as well as your body for product-free exfoliation. Just be sure to be extra gentle when rubbing it over delicate facial skin.

303 SHE'S ELECTRIC

If you have an electric toothbrush, apply cleanser to your face then use the softest bristle head to gently cleanse your face, paying extra close attention to your nose and chin.

304 FRUIT ICE SCRUB

This handy scrub should tone and make pores less visible. Chop one lemon and two apples and purée into a paste. Dispense into an ice-cube tray and freeze. Before going to bed, rub a frozen fruit cube in small circular motions on your face before moisturizing or applying a night cream.

305 NUTTY SKIN SOLUTION

If your skin looks dull and lifeless it probably needs exfoliating, so try this do-it-yourself treatment. Blend 25 g (¼ US cup) of ground almonds with 1 tablespoon of mayonnaise. Gently rub over your face and rinse well. This effective treatment may initially make your skin a little red so ideally do it before bed.

306 BRUSH AWAY

Invest in a gentle facial brush to softly scrub away dead skin cells on dry skin and you'll never have to buy an exfoliating product again.

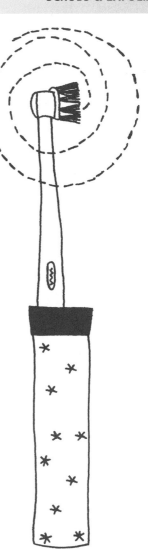

75

307 STRAWBERRY SCRUB

Strawberries contain a natural and gentle exfoliant: seeds. Mash four strawberries with a fork and mix with two tablespoons of olive oil to make a paste. Gently massage over your damp face for a moisturizing scrub.

308 SMOOTH OPERATOR

To refine pores, make an exfoliating paste by mixing a spoonful of sieved wholemeal (wholewheat) flour with a little warm water. Massage over your face and rinse for fresh, smooth feeling skin.

309 2-IN-1

Alpha Hydroxy Acids (AHAs) exfoliate the skin and unblock pores so choose a cleanser that contains AHAs and you won't need to buy a separate exfoliator.

310 MOISTURE PEEL

Use a moisturizer containing the ingredient retinol, which encourages cell turnover and unblocks pores, and you can go without a separate exfoliator.

311 A LITTLE GOES A LONG WAY

There's no need to slather exfoliator on – use too much and you could end up with sore over-scrubbed skin. A pea-sized amount is plenty for the entire face and ensures you exfoliate rather than just apply to the face. Always use gentle circular rubbing motions with the fingertips and concentrate on areas where skin cells build up, such as around the nose and chin.

312 IN THE SPHERE

A cheap exfoliator is often as good as an expensive one – just ensure the label says it contains 'beads' or 'spheres', which means the gritty, scrubbing ingredient is perfectly round. These are kinder to your skin than the uneven, rough particles which can be abrasive and harsh.

313 GIVE IT SOME FACE

Sensitive skin only needs gentle exfoliation. Rather than buying a pricy product that may upset your skin, simply exfoliate by massaging your skin with a little bit of moisturizer and a damp facecloth.

moisturizing

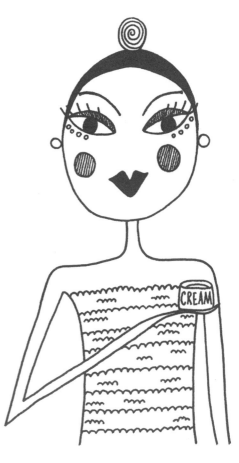

314 GET THE CREAM

Aqueous cream is often prescribed by doctors for people with dry-skin conditions and it's available in pharmacies at a fraction of the price of many branded moisturizers.

315 A-PEELING MOISTURIZER

For a money-saving smooth complexion trick, lightly wipe the inside of an avocado peeling over your clean face, using gentle, upward strokes. You can leave the oil on your face overnight or rinse off after 15 minutes.

316 CLEOPATRA'S CURE

Take a leaf out of the famous Egyptian beauty's book and bathe your skin in fresh milk for a soft, supple feel. Apply it with a cotton pad using a gentle upward motion. Leave on for a few minutes then rinse off.

317 FORGET THE SERUM

Deep-penetrating serums target specific problems and are recommended for very dry skin, but if you are getting good results from your regular moisturizer alone don't bother splashing the extra cash.

318 DISCOUNT MOISTURIZER

Many believe that an expensive moisturizer is the one product to invest in, yet the role of a moisturizer is simply to hydrate and help balance the pH. Normal skin types will flourish on a simple no-frills lotion.

319 THREE-IN-ONE

Don't splash out on a separate serum and moisturizer; look for a formula that treats as well as hydrates. If you find a formula that also contains an SPF you've eliminated the need for three separate products in a flash.

320 ADD VEGETABLE OIL

One way to make your favourite moisturizer last longer is to use a small amount of natural vegetable oil as a base first. You can also mix moisturizer with a small amount of water in the palm of your hand.

321 LITTLE GOES A LONG WAY

Overuse of moisturizer is as bad as not using any. Too much can lead to clogged pores and blackheads. A pea-sized amount should be enough for your whole face.

322 DO-IT-YOURSELF FACE CREAM

You can make two 50 g (2 oz) jars of moisturizer by dissolving 15 g (½ oz) of beeswax into 475 ml (2 US cups) of boiled, warm water and 25 ml (⅛ US cup) of jojoba oil and 25 ml (⅛ US cup) of apricot kernel oil. Add a little more water, lemon juice and rose-water and stir until thick and opaque. Decant into a sterilized jar.

323 HYDRATE YOUR HOUSE

Central heating is very dehydrating for your skin so in the winter months it's a good idea to place a bowl of water in every room. This puts moisture back into the atmosphere and saves you spending on extra moisturizer.

324 DAY AND NIGHT CREAM

Separate moisturizers for day and night are a great marketing gimmick but you only really need one cream for your skin type. Normal to oily skin types are fine with day cream, while people with dry skin can use a richer night cream for both day and night.

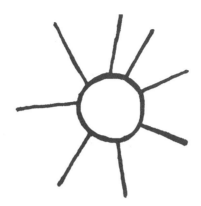

325 CHECK THE SPF

Protection from the sun is vital to prevent premature ageing of the skin so ensure that your moisturizer has a high SPF factor. You'll also save some money as you won't have to buy an expensive facial sunscreen.

326 MIX YOUR OWN TINT

You can spend a fortune on tinted moisturizers that promise to produce a 'natural glow' but if you mix some leftover bronzing powder together with your last bit of sunscreen you can make summer last longer and have a protective SPF built in too.

327 MAKE YOUR OWN OIL

Steal a trick from aromatherapy and make your own facial oil with 100 ml (½ US cup) of base oil such as macadamia nut, rose hip or evening primrose. Then mix in a few drops of an essential oil such as lavender for normal skin, sandalwood for oily skin or rose for dry and mature skin.

328 APPLY AT THE RIGHT TIME

You will need less moisturizer and it will be much more effective if you apply it at the right time. Don't wait for your skin to feel dry, apply moisturizer immediately after you wash or shower while the skin is still damp, to seal in the moisture.

329 TARGET AREAS

Another way to make moisturizer last longer is to only apply it to those parts of the face that really require hydration. For most people it's the forehead and cheeks that tend to be drier, while the chin rarely needs any extra moisture.

anti-ageing

330 PAY FOR BRIGHTENING

Look for day creams with added facial-brightening ingredients to increase the product's anti-ageing effect. They help skin reflect flattering pink tones of light and add a luminescent glow to the face.

331 VINEGAR VANISH

Vinegar is a great treatment for age spots. Mix equal parts onion juice and vinegar. Test a little on your wrist first to check for allergies. Apply every day to age spots using cotton balls. It will take a few weeks to work, but it's worth persevering as so do expensive products.

332 JOIN THE A-LIST

To fight wrinkles effectively make sure any cream you buy contains some form of vitamin A. Often listed as retinoids, these have been clinically proven to reduce the appearance of lines, increase cell turnover and improve skin texture.

333 CABBAGE MASK

This mask will counteract wrinkles and dryness and give your skin a healthy bloom thanks to the natural healing chemicals in this leafy veg. Grind two cabbage leaves to extract the juice. Dissolve a pinch of yeast into the liquid and stir in 1 teaspoon of honey. Apply thickly and leave on for 15 minutes before removing.

334 FINGER-TAP MASSAGE

Tapping quickly and lightly all along your facial bone structure helps the lymphatic nodes to drain any congested areas and eliminates toxins. Much cheaper than paying for a facial.

335 POMMIE PUNCH

There's no need to buy an expensive anti-ageing skin serum. Pomegranate oil contains a high number of antioxidants and can be found cheaply in most health-food stores. Antioxidants fight ageing by stimulating cell regeneration and minimizing the appearance of wrinkles. Use at night for maximum benefits.

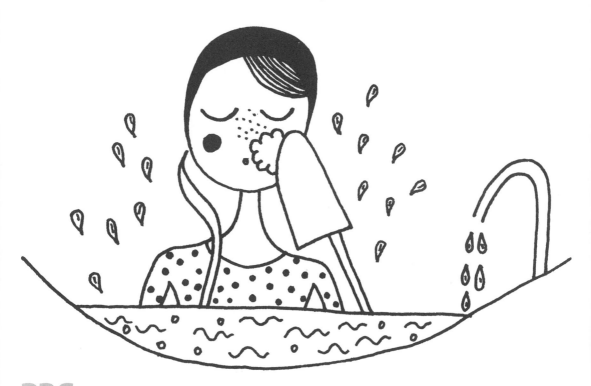

336 JUST ADD WATER

Applying anti-ageing products to slightly damp skin helps kickstart the products' active ingredients. Not only will they start work straight away, they'll also penetrate the outer layer of the skin more easily so you really get your money's worth.

337 CHECK WHAT'S WORKING

So you're spending a small fortune on several miracle face creams, but do you know what's actually working? Cut back on what you're using and test each product for a few weeks to see which is most effective. Save your money for those.

338 AND BREATHE...

Boost the effectiveness of your night cream by taking three deep breaths in and out before you apply. This will boost the levels of oxygen to the skin.

339 DON'T OVERLOAD

Layering too many products on top of each other (think serum, moisturizer, eye cream) can overload skin and cause irritation. Save money by paring down your routine.

340 STOP THE SAGGING

The main reason facial muscles sag is a lack of muscular exercise. Regular massage for a few minutes a day is a free and effective preventative. Simply make circular motions with your palm heel evenly around your face.

do-it-yourself facials

341 SET THE MOOD

Light a scented candle and play some soft music to recreate that special spa feel in your own bathroom so you can get the maximum relaxation benefits.

342 CLEAN UP

First remove make-up and cleanse the face. You can use soap and water or whatever cleanser you prefer to use. Cleansing the skin first is an important step to any facial. Gently pat skin dry after cleansing and rinsing.

343 REVITALIZE TIRED SKIN

To mimic an expensive salon treatment, stock up on the right products. Wash your face with a cleanser that contains vitamin C to enhance radiance, massage with an oxygenating serum and moisturize with a cream containing antioxidants such as vitamins E and C and pomegranate extract.

344 GET STEAMY

Gently heat enough distilled water to fill a shallow wide bowl, adding skin-friendly herbs such as rosemary, camomile or calendula. With a towel over your head, place your face over the bowl (a safe distance away so as not to damage your skin) and steam for five minutes to loosen dirt.

345 MAKE A COMPRESS

Use some of the cooled but still-warm water from the steam bowl to make a compress. Add a few drops of lavender oil for normal to dry skin and tea tree oil for congested skin. Drench a facecloth in the relaxing aromatic mixture and press it against your face five to ten times while you relax.

346 EYE SOOTHER

Apply a rich eye cream under each eye and a smear of petroleum jelly on the lips to soak in and treat the areas while the compress works. The warmth will ensure the moisture is absorbed better.

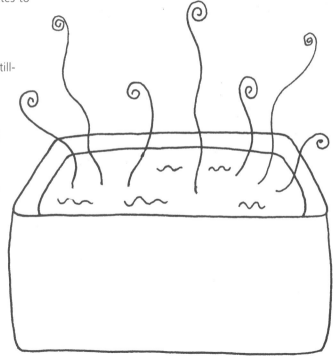

347 REVEAL A FRESHER FACE

Many microdermabrasion kits feature at-home versions of fine crystal exfoliants used by dermatologists and beauty salons, but at a do-it-yourself price. Exfoliation helps to improve skin by removing the dead skin cells. Follow the manufacturer's directions carefully, and steer clear if you have sensitive skin.

348 SPRAY AWAY

Fill a clean, sterilized spray bottle with herbal tea or lavender water and keep stored in the refrigerator for one week. Spray on to tone and close the pores after applying a compress (see tip 345).

349 RUB IN GOODNESS

To soothe the skin in the last phase of a facial, an oil or serum should be massaged into the skin. Put a generous amount onto your hands and work them together to warm up the cream. Concentrate on areas where muscles are overworked – cheeks, mouth and forehead.

face masks

350 MAKE YOUR OWN MUD PACK

You can buy large bags of deep-sea mud from most health-food stores for a tiny cost. Mix 2 cups of the mud with a cup of water to form the basis of an effective mud pack – great for drawing oil and other impurities from the skin.

351 SUB-LIME SKIN

For a deep cleanser, whisk together 2 teaspoons of olive oil and ½ teaspoon of lime juice. Cover your face with a thin layer of the mixture and leave on for 30 minutes. You'll be amazed how much dirt this lifts when you wipe it off with a dry cloth.

352 FEELING FRUITY?

This is a great treatment to soften and brighten all skin types. Mash a banana and add the juice of a pear. Mix with 2 tablespoons of natural (plain) yogurt to make a creamy paste and apply to your skin. Leave for 20 minutes, then rinse well.

353 PRETTY POPPY

Poppy seeds contain natural oils that can help nourish and moisturize dry skin. Soak 50 g (1/3 US cup) poppy seeds in water overnight, then grind them using a pestle and mortar. Add a little milk to form a paste. Apply to your face, leave on until it dries and then rinse.

354 HYDRATING HONEY

Rub 2–3 tablespoons of manuka honey onto your face and leave for about 20 minutes to enable this everyday kitchen ingredient to work its double magic – killing bacteria and moisturizing deeply. Rinse with warm water and pat dry with a towel and you should be left with clear, plump skin.

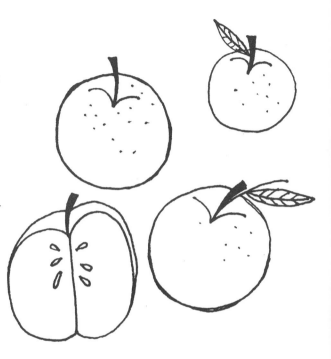

355 BLUEBERRY DELIGHT

This homemade mask contains natural antioxidants and vitamins to revive tired skin. Mix 40 g (1/4 US cup) mashed ripe blueberries with 2 tablespoons of natural (plain) yogurt. Apply the mixture to clean skin. Once it has dried, rinse off with warm water.

356 APPLE-A-DAY KEEPS ACNE AWAY

Apple is a key ingredient for a blemish-free complexion. Mix equal amounts of grated apple and honey. Clean your face then apply the apple and honey mixture. Leave on for ten minutes, then rinse with cool water.

357 GREAT GRAPES

This simple mask will smooth the appearance of fine lines. Take a bunch of green, seedless grapes and crush to a fine pulp. Add 2 tablespoons of flour to make a paste. Apply to face and allow to sit on skin for 15 to 20 minutes. Then rinse.

358 THE BREAKFAST CLUB

This homemade mix works well on dull or pale skin. Mash the flesh of one tangerine. Add 4 tablespoons of softened cream cheese and mix. Apply the fruity paste to your face and rest for ten minutes before rinsing. To make it even more economical, spread any leftovers on your breakfast bagel!

359 ASPIRIN APPLICATION

To reduce inflammation and brighten dull skin, mash between six and ten uncoated aspirins using the back of a spoon and mix with a little moisturizer. Apply to your face, let the mixture dry completely, then rinse off with warm water, rubbing in small circles to gently exfoliate.

360 COCO-LOCO

Try the following cure for sore or sunburnt skin. Beat an egg and add 2 tablespoons of coconut oil and 1 of honey. Whisk until smooth. Spoon the mixture into an empty cardboard kitchen (paper towel) roll and freeze overnight. Peel back the cardboard and apply the soft, frozen mush to your skin. Leave it on for five to ten minutes before washing off.

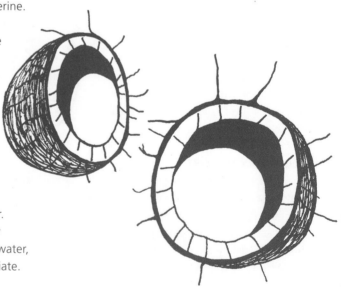

361 GELATINE PEEL

A tablespoon of plain gelatine powder plus ½ cup of fruit juice is the basis for any salon-standard gel mask. Heat in the microwave to dissolve the gelatine then put in the refrigerator to set. Citrus juices are best for oily skin while apple juice is good for drier skins.

362 FIRM FAVOURITE

This do-it-yourself mask is great for firming skin and can be made with milk, water, or cooled green tea for extra antioxidants. Add 1–2 tablespoons of kaolin powder to just enough liquid to achieve a fine paste, adding the powder teaspoon by teaspoon. Apply with your fingers and leave on for 10–12 minutes. Rinse well with warm water.

363 PERKY PEACH

Peaches contain alpha-hydroxy acids that remove dull, dead skin to reveal a fresher skin layer beneath. Cook a peach until it's soft, mash with a fork, add a tablespoon of honey and some oatmeal. Apply and leave on for ten minutes before rinsing.

364 MOISTURIZING MAYONNAISE

The ultimate deep moisturizer for dry skin is ordinary mayonnaise. Apply generously to your face and leave for three to five minutes; rinse off and follow up with a little warm olive oil to lock in the moisture.

365 TROPICAL ACNE TREATMENT

The fruit enzymes found in papayas aid the healing of skin disorders such as acne. Purée fresh pineapple and papaya in a blender. Add 1 tablespoon of honey and blend until smooth. Apply this home-prepared mask to the face and leave on for 15 to 20 minutes. Rinse off, or remove with a damp facecloth, and pat dry.

366 EGG-WHITE MASK

This simple mask is great for oily skin. Simply whisk an egg white until stiff and then add 6 drops of lemon juice and 6 drops of witch hazel. Apply to the face and leave for 15 minutes until it is tight and dry before rinsing off with lots of warm water.

remedies for common problems

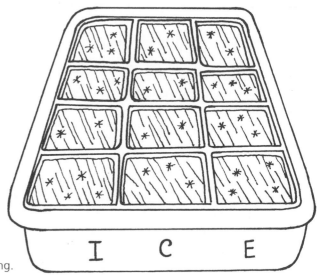

367 BIG FREEZE

There's no need to apply expensive spot (pimple) treatments. Put a few spoonfuls of parsley flakes into an ice-cube tray, add water and freeze overnight. Wrap the ice cube in a paper towel and hold for 20 seconds on your spot (pimple). This should quickly take down the swelling.

368 DO-IT-YOURSELF PORE-CLEANSING STRIPS

Make your own pore-cleansing strip by mixing 1 part unflavoured powdered gelatine with 1½ parts milk. Heat in the microwave for ten seconds, until slightly warm. Apply to your nose and chin using a cotton bud (swab). Allow the mixture to dry for 10 to 15 minutes, until it forms a stiff strip. Then peel it off.

369 A SPOT OF TOOTHPASTE

To dry spots (pimples) out simply dab toothpaste on them before you go to bed. Make sure you allow enough time for the toothpaste to dry before going to sleep to avoid smearing it on your pillow. Don't try this with sensitive skin or it could leave a red mark. It's best to test first.

370 GENERAL APPLICATION

Spot (pimple) treatments are usually simply antibacterial lotions. So why spend a lot on a branded formulation when you can achieve similar results by applying a general antiseptic cream to your blemish with a cotton bud (swab)? Try your ordinary first-aid cream first.

371 AWAKENING AVOCADO

Slice a peeled avocado into crescent shapes. Place a few slices under each eye and leave for 20 minutes. It's worth the wait, as this fabulous fruit will not only soothe tired eyes but it will also reduce puffiness following a big night out.

372 APPLE IT

Apple's natural acidity reduces inflammation. Peel an apple, cut it into small chunks and soak in boiling water for about five minutes until it turns crumbly. Drain and leave to cool until just warm. Then press the mixture onto the spot (pimple) to draw out the redness. You can also add honey to turn it into a face mask.

373 BERRY GOOD BLEMISH ZAPPER

Rather than buying expensive treatments to target that troublesome spot (pimple) on your chin, cut a strawberry in half and rub it onto the blemish. The acidic juices will open up pores and thoroughly cleanse the area.

374 GREEN SOOTHES RED

Sunburnt skin can be soothed and inflammation reduced using the wonder cure – green tea. Simply soak a facecloth in chilled green tea for instant relief.

375 JUST ADD VINEGAR

Give your regular hand cream a boost by mixing in an equal part of ordinary vinegar – this will create an effective solution for chapped and sore skin.

376 BANISH RED EYE

The inexpensive, and aptly named, herb eyebright is known to reduce redness and soothe irritated eyes. Steep 2 tablespoons of the tincture in hot water and when cooled, dip in a cotton ball and wipe over eyelids. Never use the tincture directly in the eye.

377 HERBAL RELIEF

Fennel tea that has steeped for five minutes and cooled is an effective and cheap way to reduce swelling and puffiness. Wipe the eyes with this solution several times a day.

378 DETOX TEA

Toxins in the body are the cause of many skin problems, including rashes and acne. Sipping tea made from nettle and mint can help eliminates toxins, regulate hormones and ease inflammation.

379 BRIGHT EYES

Refrigerated cucumber slices will reduce puffiness around your eyes if left on for ten minutes. Potato peelings also have the same effect; apply the moist side of fresh peels to your skin and leave on for 15 minutes.

380 BRILLIANT BAG BANISHER

Some eye gels cost enough to break the bank and promise all sorts of miracles. Save your pennies and combat dark circles with a fresh fig. Simply cut it in two and place one half over each eye for a few minutes.

381 TEATIME FOR TIRED EYES

Tea is great for reducing the appearance of puffiness and dark circles. After making two cups of tea, place the used tea bags in the refrigerator. Lie down and place a chilled tea bag over each eye.

382 SORE-EYE SOOTHER

For tired or bloodshot eyes, soak cotton balls in cold skimmed milk. Place over your eyes for ten minutes. Rinse face with warm, then cool, water.

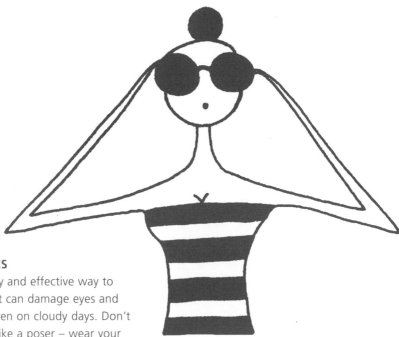

383 STAY IN THE SHADES

Sunglasses are an easy and effective way to block the UV rays that can damage eyes and cause crow's-feet – even on cloudy days. Don't worry about looking like a poser – wear your sunnies all year round.

384 COLD-SPOON COMPRESS

Cold compresses are great for combating dark circles. Place two spoons under cold, running water and then press them against your tired eyes. This treatment is just as effective as a store-bought, gel eye mask.

385 SKIP THE CREAM

Despite claims made by skincare companies, there's no difference in the active ingredients for an under-eye cream and your normal moisturizer, so unless the skin under your eyes is drier than the rest of your face, give eye cream a miss.

healthy hair

386 PRE-SHAMPOO BOOSTER

There's no need to spend a fortune on the pre-shampoo treatments that hairstylists try to sell you these days. Brushing your dry hair thoroughly before showering should remove product build-up and help stimulate the scalp to promote blood flow, which in turn delivers strengthening nutrients to hair follicles.

387 HAIR-MAXIMIZING MASSAGE

Rather than relying on products, get right to the root of the problem yourself. Massaging your scalp with small circular motions every day using your fingertips will boost blood circulation to your hair follicles, stimulating growth and shine.

388 HEALTHY HATS

The sun has a damaging effect on your hair, but expensive SPF sprays aren't the answer. Simply invest in a hat that offers UV protection.

389 FREE HAIR SHINE

Rinsing is the best shine-enhancing treatment for your hair – and costs nothing. A good rinse ensures the hair cuticles lie flat so that they can reflect maximum light. For the ultimate gloss, grin and bear water as cold as you can stand for two minutes.

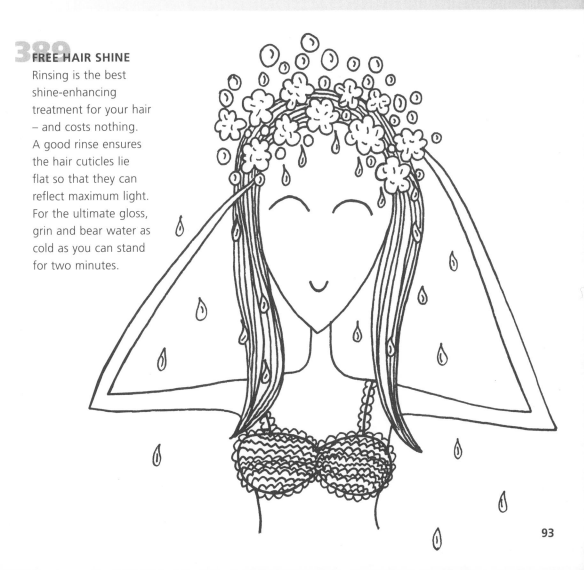

380 COCO HYDRATION

Damaged hair can be porous, and will absorb chemicals and moisture unevenly. Moisture can be replaced with conditioning treatments but don't head to the salon or pharmacy. Instead, apply warmed coconut oil to dry mid-lengths and the ends of your hair. Wrap your hair in a towel and sit in a steamy environment for 20 minutes before shampooing twice to remove oil.

381 DANDRUFF-BUSTING RINSE

For shiny, dandruff-free hair at a head-turning price, add a tablespoon of apple cider vinegar to a glass of tepid water. Pour it over shampooed hair and massage into your scalp before rinsing.

382 SCENT-SATIONAL STYLE

Put a few drops of an old perfume in a bottle with distilled water. Shake the bottle and spritz onto your hair to revive and freshen it after a night out or a day at the office. Or, for a stronger freshening effect, spray perfume directly onto a brush, then gently brush through your hair.

383 POMEGRANATE POWER

Pomegranate oil is a salon-standard hot-oil treatment. Simply heat in warm water and apply to your hair before shampooing to soothe and condition. Pomegranate oil will enhance the appearance and feel of your hair, help with detangling and moisturize the hair shaft.

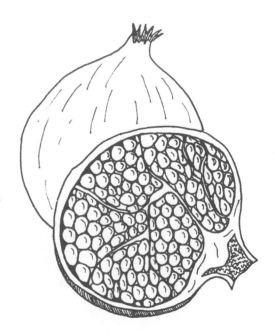

394 BUILD-UP BUSTER

Pollution, hair products and even shampoos can cause build-up on your hair and leave it looking dull. Instead of using an expensive specialist shampoo, clear build-up using a simple vinegar rinse. After shampooing, soak your hair with a solution made from three parts water, one part vinegar, then rinse thoroughly.

395 POOL PROTECTION

You don't have to buy an expensive product to protect your hair from harsh chemicals at the swimming pool. Simply comb your usual conditioner through damp hair before hitting the pool, then rinse and shampoo as normal post-swim.

396 DITCH ANTI-DANDRUFF

Many store-bought dandruff treatments contain tea tree oil. So cut out the middleman and buy your own tea tree oil. Massage it into your scalp after shampooing to help clear dandruff and soothe an itchy scalp. A little will go a long way so a small bottle will last months.

397 NOURISHING NETTLE

Nettle tea boosts circulation and hair growth while adding shine, and is available at health-food stores for a reasonable price. Brew half a cup, allow to cool and then massage into your scalp. Leave for five minutes, then rinse.

398 DANGEROUS DRYING

Wet hair can be damaged easily, so leave all styling until it is completely dry and you'll save money on electric dryers and heat-protection products. Squeeze the water out of your hair using your hands and then use a towel to gently blot. Let your hair dry naturally.

399 BEER BENEFITS

If your hair is prone to frizz, rinse with leftover flat beer after shampooing. It leaves hair full-bodied and glistening as the proteins from the hops and malt help repair and protect. Rinse thoroughly with warm water. Don't worry about smelling like a brewery – the boozy scent won't be as noticeable once your hair's dry!

shampoo & condition

400 SPIRIT CLEANSING

Any kind of alcoholic drink will have a drying effect when applied to oily hair. The higher the alcohol content, the better the effect. Mix a shot glass of vodka, or whatever spirit you have, with a couple of cups of water and rinse through your hair.

401 SAVE ON SHAMPOO

Washing your hair every day can strip away the natural oils that help protect the hair and keep it looking and feeling healthy. Try washing your hair every second or third day to maintain a natural moisture balance and save on shampoo.

402 CONDITIONING COCONUT

Many shampoos for dry hair contain coconut, so why not make your own? Simply add a few drops of coconut oil to your ordinary shampoo and use as normal.

403 DO-IT-YOURSELF DEEP CONDITIONING

There's no need to head to the salon for a deep-conditioning treatment. To intensify the effects of a home conditioner, give your hair a quick blast with a hairdryer after applying. The heat will open the cuticles allowing the ingredients to penetrate the hair shaft more deeply.

404 DRY-HAIR NOURISHER

Glycerine is the best ingredient you can use to give your shampoo extra moisturizing power. Bottles of this clear liquid can be bought from pharmacies. Mix a little with your shampoo in the palm of your hand to give your hair incredible softness and protect it from the drying effects of styling.

405 BE AN EGGHEAD

Run out of shampoo? Beat two eggs in a cup of warm water. Add a squirt of lemon juice if you have oily hair. Massage the mixture through your hair, leave on for ten minutes then rinse with warm water. Make sure the water isn't too hot or you'll end up with scrambled egg on your head!

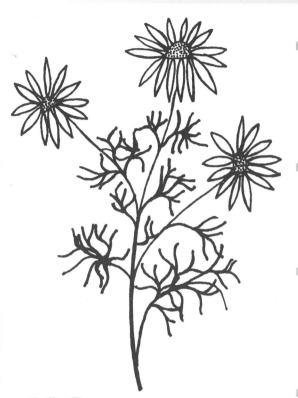

407 MOOD BOOSTER

Transform ordinary shampoo into a sensual experience by mixing in a few drops of essential oils. Lavender can transform your shower into a soothing experience, while peppermint invigorates.

408 ROSE WATER FOR SUPER SHINE

Instead of buying a pricey, perfumed shampoo, add a few drops of rose water to any basic product and your hair will smell amazing, plus it will impart incredible shine.

409 SHAMPOO STRETCHER

If you can't give up your favourite expensive shampoo, make it last longer. Put a bit of bicarbonate of soda (baking soda) in your hand with a small blob of shampoo, then lather up for more froth with less product.

410 IGNORE AD POWER

Found a product that works for you? Then stick with it rather than hankering after the latest 'miracle' product. If you do fancy a change try free samples – from magazines or direct from the brand's website – first.

406 COLOUR CODING

Turn no-frills shampoo into a bespoke product. Add a cooled cup of camomile tea to enhance blonde hair and boiled and strained rosemary leaves for brunettes.

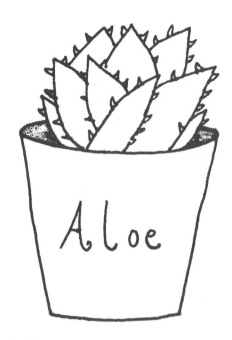

411 THE ULTIMATE
HOMEMADE CONDITIONER

Mix 60 ml (generous ¼ US cup) of almond
oil and 4 tablespoons of aloe vera gel with
10 drops of rosemary essential oil. The oil
softens, aloe hydrates, while rosemary adds
body and is a great remedy for itchy scalps.

412 READ THE LABEL

Expensive shampoos and conditioners
are rarely better than their economical
counterparts. In fact, many use the
same ingredients. Always compare the
ingredients listed on an expensive product
with the ingredients of a cheaper version.

413 GOING TO NEW LENGTHS

Emulsify shampoo and conditioner in your
hands with a little warm water before
applying to your hair. That way it will
spread further and you will use less.

414 LESS IS MORE

Only use a small amount of conditioner.
Too much of it can cause your hair to
become lank and heavy, and you'll feel the
need to wash it more often.

415 BEAUTY SLEEP

Another way to intensify the effects of your
usual conditioner is to leave it on overnight.
Wrap your hair in cling film (plastic wrap)
to protect the pillows. You'll wake with
thoroughly hydrated hair.

416 CARROT-TOP CONDITIONER

Instead of buying a conditioner formulated for oily hair, simply massage finely grated carrots into your wet hair for 15 minutes before rinsing.

417 CREAM OF THE CROP

Substitute condensed milk for your regular conditioner. Simply massage in as normal, then rinse out for a super shiny mane.

do-it-yourself hair masks

418 BE A GREEN GODDESS

Avocado contains natural oils and vitamins B6 and E, which are often found in expensive haircare products. For soft, silky locks mash half an avocado with 2 teaspoons of natural (plain) yogurt and 1 teaspoon of olive oil. Massage the mixture into your hair and leave on for ten minutes before rinsing.

419 OIL FIX

For oily hair, mix 5 tablespoons natural (plain) yogurt with 1 tablespoon bicarbonate of soda (baking soda) and 1 tablespoon fresh lemon juice. Apply the mixture to your hair, concentrating on the roots, and leave it on for 40 minutes before rinsing out.

420 DANDRUFF BUSTER

Mix one glass of red wine with five cloves of dandruff-fighting garlic and 1 tablespoon of vegetable oil. Place the mixture in a microwave-proof bowl. Heat for 20 seconds. Check to see that the mixture isn't too hot, then massage through your hair, from the roots to the ends, and wrap your hair in a hot towel. Let the mask penetrate for one hour and then shampoo out.

421 MAYO MAGIC

Plain mayonnaise makes a magnificent conditioning hair mask. Work a big dollop into the hair and then cover with cling film (plastic wrap) or a towel for an hour. Rinse with cool water as mayonnaise contains eggs and you don't want it to scramble!

422 THYME TO TREAT DANDRUFF

Thyme forms the base of many anti-dandruff treatments. Take a handful of leaves and boil in 1 litre (4 US cups) of water. Leave to cool overnight before straining and adding 2 teaspoons of apple cider vinegar or lemon juice. Massage into the scalp and leave the mixture on for at least 15 minutes before shampooing.

423 SPLIT END FIX

This treatment helps to smooth down split ends, plus it adds body and shine. Massage 3 tablespoons of warm olive oil into your scalp and hair. Cover your hair with a shower cap and leave on for at least 30 minutes before shampooing as usual.

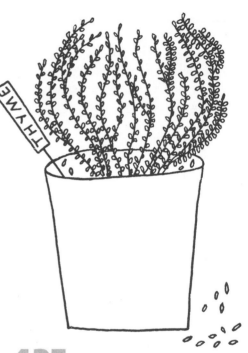

424 RUM REMEDY

This nourishing treat is especially good for adding shine to dark hair. Mix 1 tablespoon of rum and 1 tablespoon of brewed, cooled black tea. Apply the mixture to your hair, starting at the roots. Leave the mask to penetrate deeply into your hair for 30 minutes, then shampoo out.

425 HYDRATING HONEY

For shiny, nourished hair, mix 2 tablespoons of honey with 1 tablespoon of olive oil and 1 tablespoon of apple cider vinegar. Apply the mixture to your roots and then use a comb to distribute it to the ends. Leave the mask on for an hour, then rinse.

426 THICKENING MASK

For a good thickening mask mix 1 tablespoon of oat flakes with 1 tablespoon of castor oil or almond oil and 1 tablespoon of milk. Apply the mixture to your hair, working through from the roots to the ends. Leave the mask on for at least an hour, then rinse thoroughly.

427 SMOOTHIE MASK

Blend half a banana with a quarter of a melon, a quarter of an avocado, 1 tablespoon of natural (plain) yogurt and 1 tablespoon of wheatgerm oil. Leave on for 15 minutes, then rinse. This mask will leave your hair feeling soft and static-free.

428 SPLITTING HAIRS

This mask will help make split ends easier to manage. Mix 2 tablespoons of honey with 1 tablespoon of mashed avocado and 1 tablespoon of almond oil. Apply to your hair, concentrating on the ends. Leave for 30 minutes, then rinse.

429 BERRY GOOD SHINE

This mix of rich acidic berries and creamy mayo leaves hair conditioned and glossy. Mash eight strawberries with 1 tablespoon of mayonnaise. Massage into washed, damp hair. Cover with a shower cap, then a warm towel. Leave on for 20 minutes before washing out.

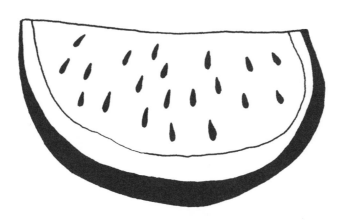

430 PERFECT PARSLEY

To restore the natural health of heat-damaged hair, pour boiling water over a handful of parsley, strain and mix with a tablespoon of vodka and a little sesame oil. Allow to cool until just warm. Rub the mixture into the roots of your hair and wrap your head in a hot towel for one hour. Rinse thoroughly and follow with a mild shampoo.

431 DAIRY QUEEN

Natural (plain) yogurt can be used to both soothe an itchy scalp and help cure dandruff. Apply, wrap your hair in a towel and then rinse after 15 minutes.

432 POTATO HEAD

To help beat thinning hair, peel and blend one potato. Mix 2 tablespoons of the potato juice from the blender with 2 tablespoons of aloe vera gel and 1 tablespoon of honey. Rub the mixture into your roots and massage into the scalp. Cover your hair with a shower cap or towel. Wash off after one hour.

cuts

433 DO-IT-YOURSELF BLUNT FRINGE (BANGS)

Save on cost and cut your own fringe (bangs). Always cut when your hair is dry. Section off the hair you don't want to cut and tie it back. Comb your fringe (bangs) down. Rest the comb on your brow bone with the teeth facing out. Don't cut your fringe (bangs) any shorter than where the comb hits your face. Start 'point-cutting' – snipping at a 45-degree angle. Never cut straight across as it's impossible to keep to a perfectly straight line.

434 DO-IT-YOURSELF LONG FRINGE (BANGS)

Tie the rest of your hair back in a ponytail. Use a brand-new, disposable single-blade razor instead of scissors. Pull your fringe (bangs) taut between your middle and index fingers. Slide fingers all the way down to the end of your hair and then razor-cut the hair just above your fingers.

435 BOB IT

A style that has very little layering or is all one length, like a bob or crop, is stylish and will keep its shape as it grows, making frequent trims unnecessary. A chin-length bob will still look good when it has grown to your shoulders – which means about six months between haircuts!

436 SHORT OF CASH

Short, layered styles need a lot of maintenance to keep them looking good. Longer haircuts have more versatility and can be worn tied up as the style grows out. If you're going for a short chop ask your stylist for a cut that will grow out well so you don't have to return too soon.

437 HAIR-CUTTING CLASSES

Cutting your own hair is risky if you don't know what you're doing. Next time you visit the hair salon, ask about local hair-cutting classes or look them up on the internet. You'll have to pay for the course, but if you stick to simple styles it could save you a fortune in hairstylist's bills in time.

438 LOW-COST LAYERS

Ask for a few longer layers to frame your face. This is cheaper than a completely layered style, and it should maintain its shape while growing out so you won't have to visit the salon as often.

439 BUDGET FOR YOUR HAIR

If you are going to spend money on just one thing to keep your hair looking beautiful, make it the haircut. A great haircut will give you a polished look, whatever products you use.

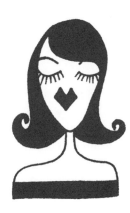

colour & highlights

440 SEAL DYE WITH VINEGAR

Rinse just-dyed hair with diluted white vinegar as a final rinse. This seals your colour so it won't fade as quickly and you can wait longer between treatments.

441 MIX AND MATCH

For a more unique look, mix two shades (it's a good idea to stick to the same brand) to create your own colour. Go for darker tones on the layers underneath and lighter ones at the top and front of your hair.

442 SINKING IN

Mist the ends of your hair with water before home-colouring. The ends of your hair are more porous and, as a result, absorb more pigment. Wet hair doesn't absorb colour as readily as dry hair. This will help you achieve an even colour while using less product.

443 GET A PROFESSIONAL OPINION

If you're thinking about dyeing your hair, pop into the hair salon and chat to them about what colours would suit you. After they've given you their thoughts, say that you're going to think about it and then go home and do it yourself.

444 HOME HELP

While highlights can be complicated, covering up grey hair or trying a new all-over colour is easy to do yourself. Home-dye kits are now hydrating and user-friendly. The key to dyeing your hair at home is to only go one or two shades darker or lighter, and no more.

445 ROOT TOUCH UP

To touch up your roots at home, start at your hairline and, using a brush applicator, brush the dye into the roots, being careful not to miss any areas. Divide the rest of your hair into sections and brush the dye into your roots along these sections. Getting a friend to help will make doing the back of your head easier.

446 SAVVY SHAMPOOING

If you dye your hair, a great money-saving idea is to always use shampoos that are designed for colour-treated hair. You'll cut down on how frequently you need to re-dye because these shampoos are designed not to strip the colour.

447 NATURAL HIGHLIGHTS

Sun exposure lightens your hair naturally and you can heighten the effects by squirting your hair with lemon juice and letting it dry in the sun. This can be very drying for your hair, though, so follow exposure with deep-conditioning home treatments.

448 COLOUR REJUVENATOR

Coloured hair can become dull. To breathe life back into your coloured hair, mix a couple of tablespoons of apple cider vinegar with a jug of warm water. After shampooing, pour the rinse over your head, massage in thoroughly and rinse out. Repeat every couple of weeks and your hair should retain its colour and shine.

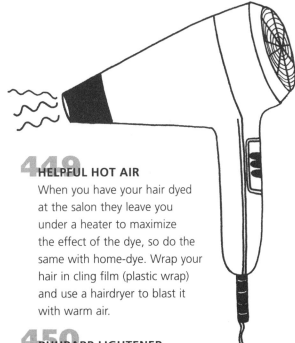

448 HELPFUL HOT AIR

When you have your hair dyed at the salon they leave you under a heater to maximize the effect of the dye, so do the same with home-dye. Wrap your hair in cling film (plastic wrap) and use a hairdryer to blast it with warm air.

450 RHUBARB LIGHTENER

For a natural lightening effect, simmer 4 tablespoons of powdered rhubarb root in 700 ml (1½ US pt) of water for 30 minutes, steep for several hours, strain, then rinse through your hair several times. Rhubarb root can be purchased from health food stores and Chinese herbalists.

451 GO SEMI-NATURAL

Maintaining a bleached blonde look can be costly when your natural colour is more mousey than Scandinavian. Try a combination of a natural brunette shade with blonde and bronze highlights for a fair look that's less high maintenance.

452 EMBRACE YOUR DARK SIDE

Many celebrities, including Madonna, Sarah Jessica Parker and Britney Spears, have proudly shown off their dark roots. You can too – just make sure the rest of your appearance is well groomed to avoid looking sloppy.

453 BEET-ROOTS

To rejuvenate red hair, mix equal amounts of beetroot (beet) juice and carrot juice. After washing your hair, pour the mixture over it, being careful of towels and walls as it will stain. Put a shower cap on your head so you don't get any on your clothes and leave for an hour before washing.

454 BLONDE TO A TEA

Bring out blonde highlights by rinsing shampooed hair with cooled camomile tea. If you have red hair, green tea is a good booster; and for grey hair, try ginseng.

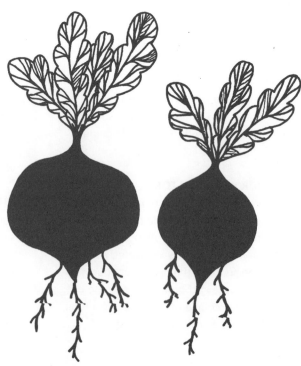

455 STICK TO THE T

If you have fine to medium-thick hair then you can ask for a partial T-section instead of getting a full head of highlights. The colourist will apply highlights just on your parting and around your face. This method is cheaper and your hair will look thicker because the darker hair underneath the highlights creates the illusion of depth.

456 HOME HIGHLIGHTS

Buy a home-highlighting kit designed for your length of hair. Those with short hair should chose one that includes a cap, while those with long hair should pick a kit that includes an application brush that lets you 'paint' on the highlights. For best results, perform highlights on completely dry, slightly dirty hair.

457 BRUNETTE BOOST

Enhance the tone and shine of brunette hair by rinsing with cold coffee. Make a pot of coffee, let it cool completely, then use it as a rinse after shampooing.

styling

458 MAKE WAVES

Wavy hairstyles make it possible to put off haircuts for longer – it's harder to see grown-out layers, dark roots or split ends.

459 NATURAL IS NICER

Use heated styling tools such as hairdryers, flat irons, curling irons and hot rollers sparingly – this will be easier if you don't wash your hair every day. Whenever possible, let your hair air-dry completely, or partially if you're pushed for time. You'll save time and money on heat-protection products – not to mention electricity!

460 ENHANCE THE SHINE

Lavender makes a great and cheap shine-enhancing hairspray. Transfer a few drops of essential oil into a spray bottle and lightly spritz onto damp hair after washing. It will smooth the cuticles and hold your style in place – and it smells gorgeous, too.

461 BETTER BRUSHSTROKES

You only really need two types of brush to style your tresses: a natural-bristled round or flat brush to use on dry hair and a soft, rubber, wide-toothed comb to use on damp hair, as it stretches and snaps more easily.

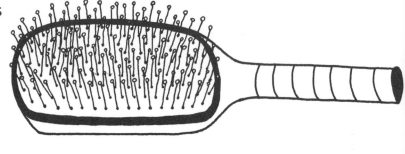

Brushes are inexpensive and it's worth shopping around as the right bristles will really help your hair appear smoother.

462 SENSIBLE BANDS

Expensive hair bands are no better for your hair than cheaper ones; just make sure they are fabric coated. Don't be tempted to use rubber bands as they can break or split hair.

463 BE A SWEETIE

Make your own hairspray: dissolve a tablespoon of sugar in a glass of hot water. Allow it to cool, pour the mixture into an old spray bottle and spritz evenly onto your hair to keep flyaways at bay.

464 GET INTO A TWIST

If your hair is naturally curly or frizzy, you can transform it into glossy ringlets at home using a little wax. While your hair is still damp, rub some wax between your fingers then take a small section of your hair and twist it around your finger. Repeat all over, for a head of fabulous curls.

465 BOOZY SHINE

Don't spend money on a shine spray – make your own. Mix beer with mineral water in a spray bottle and lightly spritz onto damp hair after washing. To disguise the smell of beer, add a drop of your favourite essential oil.

466 ELVIS-INSPIRED

If you have short hair, a quiff is a simple, funky style that you can do yourself. Simply section a 5 cm (2 inch) portion of your hair near the front and at the top of your head. Pull the hair back and then forward in a sliding motion until you get the desired height. Hold in place with hairgrips (bobby pins) and hairspray.

467 PUMP UP THE VOLUME

For a cheap body-building hairspray, mix two cups of water with the juice of one orange in a saucepan. Bring slowly to the boil then cool and strain the mixture. Pour into a spray bottle and use it on wet hair to add volume.

468 SAY 'YES' TO SURVEYS

Save money on hair products by going online. Beauty suppliers often give away free samples of shampoo, conditioners and hair dyes in return for filling out surveys or joining a mailing list.

469 LESS IS MORE

Only spritz your hair three times with hairspray. Not only is this economical but too much spray can weigh down your hair and leave it looking flat.

470 MIGHTY MOUSSE

Make your own hair mousse by beating one egg white until it forms stiff peaks. Use your fingers to rub a tiny bit of whipped egg white into your hair and then style. This trick is used by hairdressers for catwalk shows as it gives amazing hold.

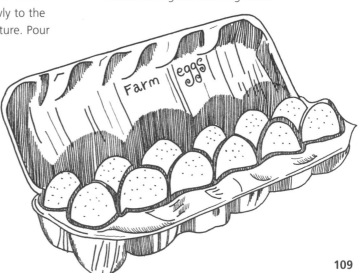

471 HOMEMADE HAIR GEL

Making your own hair gel is an easy way to save money. Dissolve ½ teaspoon of gelatine in a cup of warm water, adding more gelatine as needed to reach the desired consistency. Store in the refrigerator between uses.

472 BRUSH EXTENDER

There's no need to throw out old hairbrushes and buy new ones. Simply clean brushes by soaking them in a mild shampoo.

473 DON'T OVERDO IT

Styling products are meant for use on your hair not your head. Too much shine spray or gel will waste your product, and can cause spots (pimples) if the product gets into the pores on your face.

474 ZIG AND ZAG

If your roots are beginning to show why not put off your visit to the salon a bit longer by experimenting with a new style? Try styling your parting in a zigzag to hide your roots and make your hair look thicker.

475 TANGLE-FREE TRESSES

Run out of detangler? Fabric softener can reduce hair static to prevent tangles. Make sure you read the label first though, to ensure that it doesn't contain bleach or colouring agents. Dilute with 12 parts water and apply a little to your hair after shampooing, then rinse it off immediately.

476 FINE HAIR SOLUTION

Spend wisely and check the labels. Look out for products that contain proteins (keratin and collagen), silicone polymers or polymeric quaternium compounds. These are chemicals that stick to the hair shaft and make your hair appear thicker.

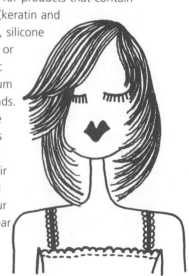

477 SWAP SHOP

If you and your mates are suckers for new products, why not get together to discuss which ones you want to try and then take turns to buy the products? This way you can all give them a go and you'll split the cost of experimenting with products that may not work for you.

478 GO THE DISTANCE

Ever wonder why professional blow-dries last longer than when you style your hair at home? The secret's in the cool air. Heat from the hairdryer opens the cuticles and allows a style to be formed, but it's the cool air that sets the style. So when you're blow-drying, finish each section with a blast of cooler air.

479 BE LABEL SAVVY

Many styling products, even the expensive ones, have alcohol as their main ingredient. These products can actually dry the hair and reduce shine. Try not to splash out on products that have alcohol listed as their first ingredient.

480 DO-IT-YOURSELF BLOW-DRY

To achieve a professional-looking blow-dry, apply a little mousse or styling lotion. Use a flat paddle brush or rounded brush while drying and finish with a spritz of serum for gloss and hairspray for hold.

481 DIVIDE AND CONQUER

When drying hair, make like your hairstylist and divide it into several manageable sections, of 5–10 cm (2–4 in) thickness. That way you can focus on styling one section and clip the rest of the hair out of the way.

482 THE STRAIGHT STORY

The hairstylist's secret for blow-drying hair straight is all about angles. To get that super-sleek look, the airflow from the blow-dryer needs to be directed down the hair shaft, from the roots towards the ends.

483 PERFECT CURLS EVERY TIME

An air diffuser is a wise investment for curly girls. Place the diffuser at the end of your blow-dryer, but stop drying while your hair still has some moisture in it to avoid frizz.

484 DO-IT-YOURSELF UPDO

Don't pay someone to put your hair up – do it yourself. Pull your hair back as if you are gathering it in a ponytail at the base of your neck. Twist in an anticlockwise (counter-clockwise) motion, then keeping your hair taut, pull it up. Use one hand to hold the twist flat against your head. Tuck the 'tail' of the hair around your fingers and underneath, securing with hairgrips (bobby pins).

485 HOME BLOW-DRY

To get a long-lasting blow-dry at home, take your time and work by sectioning your hair first. Begin with the back sections, move on to the side panels, then the fringe, top and crown. Make sure each section has been cooled before moving to the next.

486 CURL BOOSTING

Curl-boosting products can be expensive, so why not improvise? Simply rub a little of your usual conditioner between your hands then scrunch into your hair. It creates a more natural finish when dry than using mousses or gels.

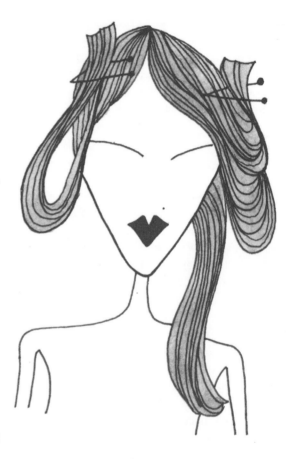

value hair treatments

487 PRICE MATCHING

Many salons will reduce the cost of your haircut if you tell them that you know you can get it cheaper across the street. Always ask if your salon will match a nearby competitor's price.

488 SAVE ON STYLISTS

If you go to a salon that offers different stylists at different prices, have your first cut and restyle with a senior stylist to ensure you get the shape and look just right then book follow-up trims with a junior stylist to save money.

489 BACK TO SCHOOL

For a big-salon cut without the big-salon price, ask if your salon has a training facility that you can visit, or enquire at a nearby hairdressing school. You'll get a discounted cut from a supervised trainee stylist.

490 DITCH THE DRYER

Leaving the salon with wet or roughly dried hair is always cheaper than letting the stylist dry and style it for you. The downside is that you don't get to see the finished look, but for long-hair trims and simple bobs it's a great way to save cash. Some salons will let you use their blow-dryers, too.

491 BRING ON THE BARBER'S

Are you a woman with a very straightforward cut? Then head to the local barber's shop. You'll pay a lot less than you would at a salon that caters solely for women, and a barber is usually just as experienced.

492 BECOME A HAIR MODEL

Willing to take risks with your hair? Then contact the top salons in your area and let them know that you're interested in becoming a hair model. You're more likely to bag a free cut if you have long hair that hasn't been chemically treated and you need to be open to a dramatic change of style and colour.

493 THINK A-HEAD

If you know your hair needs to be trimmed every six weeks it might be a wise idea to pre-book all your appointments in advance. A lot of stylists will reward your loyalty by knocking some money off your bill.

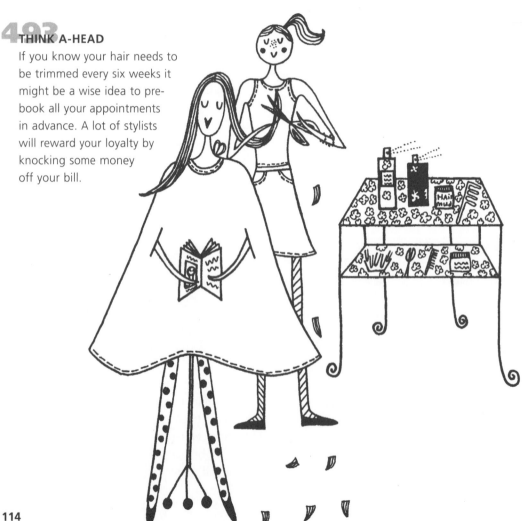

494 STRETCH IT OUT

Just because your stylist says you should come in every six weeks, that doesn't mean you have to. By lengthening the time between cuts to eight weeks you will shave two visits off of your yearly total.

495 STYLE FOR A SNIP

Plenty of high-end salons slash their prices during weekday afternoons when they're at their quietest. Don't be afraid to go inside and ask for details even if it's not advertised.

496 CHOP AND CHANGE

Save your expensive salon for a restyle. Cheaper places can handle the in-between trims by following the basic cut that's already been established.

497 IN-BETWEEN FREEBIES

Many salons offer a free in-between-appointment trim for your fringe (bangs), as this is usually the first area to grow out. Take advantage of this when all you need is a tidy-up.

498 SAVE A BUNDLE

The more treatments you have from one salon, the cheaper the price will be for the individual treatments. Instead of making separate appointments for cut, colour and manicure, book all your services for the same day. You may get a chunk off the bill or they may throw in a blow-dry for free.

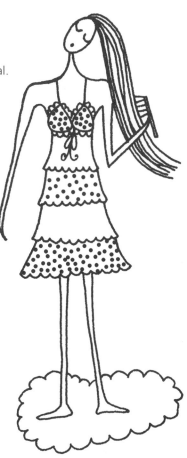

499 CHECK OUT COUPONS

Scour your local newspaper for salon vouchers. If you don't find any savings then go online. Start your search using the names of salons in your area and the word 'coupon'.

500 NEW ARRIVALS

Keep an eye out for new salons opening in your local area. They nearly always run special promotions to attract new customers. Spot one in your area and you could be rewarded with a half-price cut.

501 RESIST THE EXTRAS

It can be tempting to say 'yes' when you're offered a manicure, glass of fizz or even a sandwich, while your hair colour is developing. Don't be tempted unless you are sure it won't be added to your bill.

502 SAVE OR SPLURGE?

If you have your hair coloured professionally at a top salon, don't feel that you have to get it cut at the same time. If you've got a simple one-length style it might be worth getting it trimmed at a cheaper salon.

503 KEEP THINGS SIMPLE

The more processes you have done to your hair the more it will cost. Rather than going for highlights in several different shades, try an all-over colour gloss to bring out your natural highlights. It's easier to apply and so will cost far less.

504 FACE UP TO IT

Achieve a rich highlighted effect by requesting colour highlights (or lowlights) only around your face. Partial highlights are cheaper than a whole or half head and will make a real difference as the hair next to your face is what people notice most. Alternatively ask for 'hidden' colour, where partial-head highlights are added to underneath sections so regrow isn't obvious.

505 JUST SAY NO

Don't feel you have to buy the haircare and styling 'professional' products your hairstylist recommends; they're not going to be offended if you say no. Salon prices usually include a premium and you'll be able to get cheaper brands elsewhere.

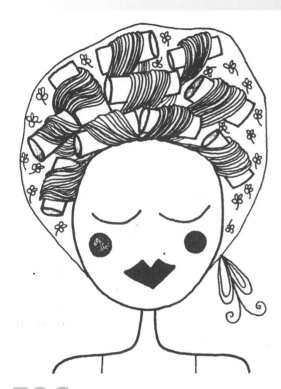

507 CUT THE COLOUR

High-maintenance colours – like light blonde or red – require frequent touch-ups that can be expensive. If you want great hair on a budget it's best to stay as close as possible to your natural colour and choose scattered highlights so that your roots are not obvious.

508 JOIN THE BRAIDY BUNCH

Can't afford to touch up dark roots? Plaiting (braiding) hair with regrowth is a favourite celebrity trick, and a great way to make a feature of the regrowth, as the contrast of colours can be striking. Any style that doesn't show the parting will hide regrowth, too, such as using hairbands or twisting the front section back to cover the crown.

509 STAGGER COLOUR

If you have a full head of highlights, save money by not getting a full colour each time your roots start to show. Use a three-visit cycle: on the first visit get the full head of highlights, then on the next two visits just get half a head.

506 STAND THE TEST OF TIME

If you can't resist getting a professional blow-dry, make it go an extra day or two by asking the stylist to use rollers instead of just a rounded brush. Drying with rollers will give a longer-lasting bounce.

hands & feet

510 ZESTY HEEL SCRUB

There's no need to buy expensive foot creams to shift rough skin on your heels. Instead, simply cut a lemon in half, squeeze out the juice and fill with sugar. Place the lemon over your heel and rub firmly.

511 TEA-RRIFIC TOOTSIES

If your feet are prone to smelling less than fragrant sometimes, there's no need to buy specialist products. The tannins in tea fight odour-causing bacteria, so to avoid stinky soles, soak your feet in cooled, strong black or green tea for several minutes before patting dry.

512 FEELING FRUITY?

To exfoliate your hands and to help reduce age spots, mix the juice of two fresh limes and 225 g (1 US cup) of sugar together. Rub into your hands, leave for three to five minutes, then rinse with warm water and pat dry.

513 FUNGUS-FREE FEET

Medicine for toenail fungus isn't cheap and doesn't always work. So treat your feet by soaking them in a mixture of equal amounts of white vinegar and water for 30 minutes daily until the condition clears.

514 BEST FOOT FORWARD

There's no need to go to the beauty salon to have a softening pedicure treatment; do it yourself. Pour 750 ml (1½ US pt) of full-fat milk into a bowl and soak your feet. It will leave your skin supersoft.

515 SMOOTHING SOCKS

Expensive moisturizers aren't the only way to fight dry, chapped skin. Mash a banana with a little honey, lemon juice and margarine to make a moisturizing paste. Smear on your feet and wear cotton socks to bed. Wash off in the morning and feel how unbelievably smooth your soles are.

516 COOL TREATMENT

Yogurt is as good as any pre-manicure conditioning treatment for hands and nails. Simply combine 225 g (1 US cup) of natural (plain) yogurt with the juice of an apple. Refrigerate for several hours and then use to massage your hands and nails. Rinse the excess off afterwards.

517 CUTER CUTICLES

If you have dry ragged cuticles, don't turn to expensive cuticle creams for help. Instead, rub leftover avocado skins into your cuticles and leave for 30 minutes. The vitamin E and natural oils in this fruit will help your fingers heal.

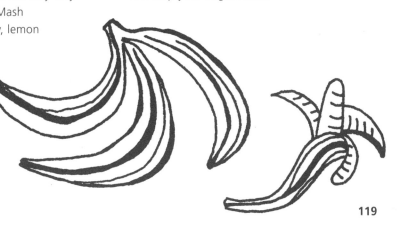

518 DOUBLE-DUTY BEAUTY

Give hands a hydrating treatment while doing the dishes. Cover them in a thick layer of moisturizer and wear dishwashing gloves. The warmth of the water will help the softening ingredients penetrate deeply, leaving you with baby-soft digits.

519 HAND RELIEF

Paying extra for lots of different lotions is a waste of money when the answer to dry hands lies in your kitchen storecupboard. Before bed, cover your hands in a generous amount of olive oil and put on cotton gloves. In the morning your hands will be softer and smoother.

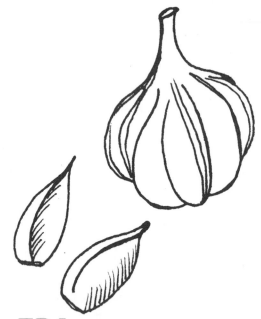

520 MILKY TIPS

For a great nail-strengthening treatment, warm a cup of milk in the microwave for 30 seconds (until warm, not boiling) and add a tablespoon of almond or sesame oil. Check the temperature of the milk to ensure it's not too hot, then massage into your hands for five minutes to strengthen nails and hydrate stressed skin.

521 HERO HERB

You can use garlic to make your nails stronger instead of expensive nail-strengthening treatments. Add 1 tablespoon of finely chopped fresh garlic to a bottle of clear nail polish. Leave the bottle for one week and then apply as needed. Don't worry – your nails won't smell and they will be far less likely to split and break.

522 JUICY SKIN SOFTENER

To make a delicious-smelling cuticle softener, blend 1 teaspoon of papaya or mango juice with ½ teaspoon of egg yolk and 1 teaspoon of cider vinegar. Apply to cuticles and leave for as long as possible before rinsing.

523 BACK TO LIFE

If your nail polish has dried up there's no need to throw it out. Just add a tiny drop of nail polish remover, shake the bottle and it's as good as new.

524 STRETCH IT OUT

You only need a little nail polish remover for it to do its job, so to make your product last longer, dampen your cotton pad with water before applying the remover. It won't soak up as much of the product.

525 SOMETHING FISHY

Cod liver oil, with its high vitamin A content will also strengthen and improve the appearance of brittle nails if you massage it into your nails at bedtime.

526 POWERFUL POMMIE HEALER

To soothe distressed fingernails and cuticles following the removal of acrylic or gel tips, soak your fingers in vitamin-rich pomegranate oil.

527 MAKE MANICURES LAST LONGER

Cleaning your nails with white vinegar before applying nail polish will create a smoother finish so your manicure will go the distance without chipping.

528 PERFECT YOUR TECHNIQUE

When applying polish you don't need to use too much – it requires just three strokes: one down the middle and one either side. Leave to dry for at least five minutes before applying a second coat. Use a cotton bud (swab) dampened with polish remover to get rid of any smudges.

529 SOLE SEARCHER

Another cost-effective way to remove hard, dead skin from your feet is to add rock salt to a little olive oil and use as a scrub. Afterwards, moisturize with warm olive oil.

530 SAVE YOURSELF FROM SPLITS

If a nail splits there is no need to pay a beauty therapist to fix it. Just buy some nail paper and fix it yourself. Cover with two coats of nail polish and the patch will be invisible.

531 TOPS AND TAILS

Don't forget to use a base coat and a top coat to make your home manicure really last. But don't spend on separate products – one bottle of clear polish will do both jobs.

532 SHAPE SHIFTER

You don't need to visit a salon to make your nails look groomed. You can make square nails appear more elegant by applying polish down the centre only. Pale shades are best for short nails or stubby hands, while darker shades make chunky hands look delicate.

533 NAIL ART NAILED

With a little practice you can apply nail art to your own nails. Once you have covered your nails in a base colour and allowed to dry, draw patterns using an old lipstick brush and a different colour of polish.

534 GET SALON SAVVY

Next time you get your nails done at a salon ask for the 'shape and polish' rather than a full manicure. They usually cost a quarter of the price and unless your cuticles are in really bad shape the end result will be identical.

535 HOME PEDICURE

It's easy to look after your toes yourself. Just remember that to prevent painful ingrowing nails, toenails should be clipped and filed straight across, never curved. Separate toes with cotton balls and apply nail polish, or buff for a natural look.

hair-removal hints

536 A CLOSE SHAVE

Don't buy shaving cream; use hair conditioner instead. To give hair a smooth, silky surface most conditioners contain silicone, which will allow the razor to slide easily over your skin for a close, nick-free shave.

537 SKIN SOOTHER

If you buy shaving cream don't waste your cash on ones that contain sodium laurel sulphate or menthol because these can dry the skin and cause irritation. Look for those with added aloe vera or glycerine for added moisture.

538 MAN, I FEEL LIKE A WOMAN

Women's razors tend to be more expensive than men's, so why not buy a men's razor? Although women's razors are probably prettier, men's ones tend to have more blades, which results in a closer shave.

539 BANISH BURN

You don't need store-bought post-shave balm to soothe razor burn. Simply rub honey onto your legs; aloe vera gel with a little witch hazel also works well.

540 PERFECT SHAVE

Forget salon waxing – shaving costs next to nothing and you avoid the horrible in-between stage of waiting for your hair to grow long enough. For the perfect leg shave, have a warm shower or bath to open your pores. Rub an exfoliator over your legs to remove dead skin. Lather up your legs and shave against the direction of hair growth. Rinse with cold water to close the pores.

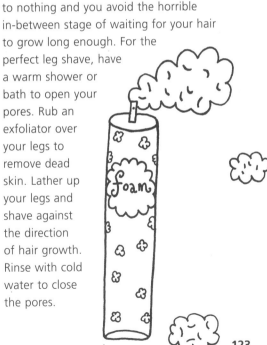

123

541 TAKE THE PAIN OUT OF WAXING

Don't waste money on numbing sprays. To minimize discomfort simply take two aspirins or ibuprofen 30–45 minutes before waxing. Then five minutes before, take a warm shower to open up the pores so that the hairs will slide out more easily.

542 MAKE YOUR OWN WAX

Stir the juice of a lemon and 50 ml (½ US cup) of water in a pan. Add 225g (1 US cup) of sugar. Heat the mixture until it thickens. When the wax turns a darker colour take it off the heat and leave to stand. Be very careful to use only when it's cool enough to be applied.

543 BIKINI MADE EASY

Nervous about waxing your own bikini line? The best wax to use is hard wax – it's made for coarse hair and 'shrink-wraps' the hairs making them easier to pull out. After waxing press your hand down on your skin to relieve pain, and use tweezers to remove any hairs missed by the wax.

544 KITCHEN KIT

Instead of buying a pre-waxing lotion try using warm water and a gentle exfoliator – just make sure to pat skin dry before waxing. And rather than buying wax remover, use baby oil or olive oil. Washed ice-lolly (ice-pop) sticks make the perfect wax applicators.

545 REVITALIZE YOUR RAZOR

Make razor blades last longer by drying the blade after use. Water that sits on blades between shaves causes rusting, which in turn causes blades to dull. By carefully blotting your razor blade on a towel, you can seriously extend its life.

546 THE OUCH-FACTOR

If you are waxing your own upper lip, you can make the experience less painful by dabbing some oral gel (the kind used to relieve the pain of mouth ulcers and denture sores) from your medicine cabinet on the area first. It numbs the skin and makes the whole process far less painful.

547 BRAVING THE COLD

Doing a perfect do-it-yourself job using cold wax is easier than you think. Simply smooth the strips onto your leg in the direction of hair growth. Hold the skin above the strip taut. Pull the strip off quickly in the opposite direction of the hair growth. It's less messy than hot waxing but just as cheap!

548 SIMPLE SUGARING

Sugaring gets just as good results as waxing, but it's cheaper, easier and less painful. Sprinkle talcum powder on dry skin. Apply the sugaring paste thinly in the direction of hair growth. Press on a strip of paper and pull it off against the direction of hair growth.

549 DABBLE WITH DEPILATORIES

Depilatory creams now contain moisturizing agents so they leave your skin extra soft and silky. The results last a lot longer than shaving, but without the cost of professional hair removal.

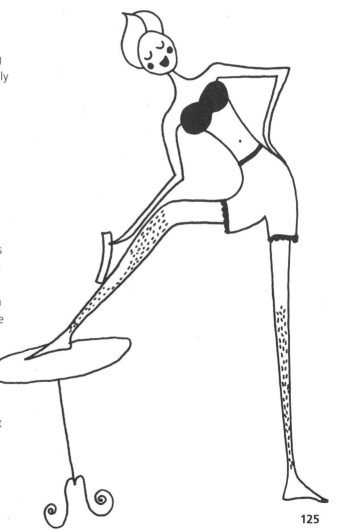

550 WISE WARM-UP TIPS

When waxing at home it's important to prepare properly. Exfoliate first, then wet the skin with warm water and leave for five minutes. This opens the hair follicles and thickens the hair as it absorbs the water, which will help the wax stick to it.

551 SKIN SOOTHER

Don't waste money on after-wax cream or lotion – many contain alcohol or perfume that could irritate your skin. Instead, use a little tea tree oil or baby powder to soothe the skin and prevent red bumps.

552 LAVENDER SOLUTION

If your skin is sensitive or inflamed you can still beat ingrown hairs with this gentle treatment. Mix two parts sugar, to exfoliate, with one part olive oil, to moisturize. Add ten drops of tea tree oil as an antiseptic and ten drops of lavender oil as an anti-inflammatory. Rub gently in a circular motion twice a week.

553 SHOP AROUND

If you're a salon devotee, check out the cheapest electrolysis or laser hair removal prices in your area, as they can vary widely.

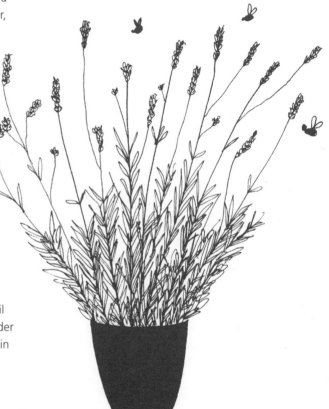

554 HAIR TODAY

Remember that hair-minimizing products are a commitment – lotions and deodorants must be used daily to be effective and the results are only typically seen after weeks of use. Only buy them if you're going to apply them religiously as otherwise there's no point spending all that money.

555 TAME TRAPPED HAIRS

Don't buy a specialist product to ease ingrowing hairs – you'll be paying a fortune for exfoliation as that is how most products work. A handful of Epsom salts rubbed onto wet skin in a circular motion will help unblock the follicle to loosen the ingrown hair (also see tip 552).

556 BY A THREAD

Threading involves wrapping a cotton thread around hairs and pulling them out from the root. It's a great alternative to plucking or waxing your eyebrows and upper lip. The results last longer and salons often charge less than they do for a professional wax.

557 BE A SWEETIE

To make your own sugaring paste, mix eight parts sugar with one part water and one part lemon juice. Heat until smooth and thick. Leave to cool until it can be spread easily and thinly.

558 HOT WAX LIKE A PRO

Apply heated wax in the direction of hair growth. Wax section by section, rather than covering the entire leg. Press the cloth strip firmly over the wax, hold your skin taut and pull off quickly.

559 WAXING LYRICAL

Don't be embarrassed by upper lip hair – be embarrassed about spending a fortune on salon waxes. For a tenth of the price you can be fuzz-free for months using a store-bought facial wax strip kit.

560 PAIN-FREE HAIR REMOVAL

Why pay for painful hair removal when you can bleach unwanted body and facial hair at home? It's easy, pain-free and affordable, plus you won't get unsightly ingrown hairs.

bag a budget brighter smile

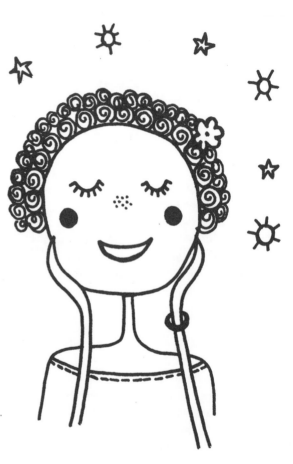

561 LEMON PEEL SMILE

Another way to achieve a white smile without spending money on bleaching products is to rub lemon peel across your teeth for a fast whitening effect.

562 BRIGHTENING BENEFITS

Lots of whitening toothpastes contain bicarbonate of soda (baking soda), so why pay for a brand name when you can achieve the same effect by simply using the product itself? Wet your toothbrush, dip it into the bicarbonate of soda (baking soda) and brush for whiter, brighter teeth.

563 PUMP IT UP

Buy toothpaste in a pump rather than a tube. You can get a pea-sized amount out of a pump so it will last longer. If you use a tube, cut the tube open to get the last bit out.

564 VANISH WITH VINEGAR

To whiten teeth and neutralize bad breath, once a week dip a wet toothbrush into white vinegar and brush your teeth. Be sure to rinse your mouth well with water afterwards, as vinegar will attack your teeth's enamel if left on too long.

565 GIVE BACTERIA THE BRUSH-OFF

To ensure your toothbrush lasts longer, always rinse it well to remove all toothpaste and food debris. Store in a well-ventilated area in an upright position to help your brush dry thoroughly. Douse with boiling water once a week to kill bacteria.

566 TOOTH SAVER

Save on dental costs by brushing properly: brush the inside and outside surfaces of your teeth using short strokes and concentrate on where the teeth meet the gums. Focus on cleaning one small area at a time. Next, brush back and forth horizontally along the chewing surfaces. Finally, lightly brush your tongue. A proper brushing routine should last three to four minutes.

567 MINTY FRESH

For instant cut-price mouthwash, mix a small amount of water with a 1/4 teaspoon of salt, a drop of tea tree oil and a drop of peppermint oil. The mixture will help eliminate bad breath and leave your mouth feeling fresh for hours.

568 MAKE WHITE LAST LONGER

If you can't resist professional whitening treatments, remember that bleaching temporarily strips away the protective coating on your teeth, making them more vulnerable to staining. To ensure the effects last longer don't eat any dark-coloured or acidic foods for at least 48 hours afterwards.

569 HALITOSIS HEALER

If gum problems are giving you bad breath, diluted tea tree oil can combat the problem better than expensive mouthwash. Mix a few drops of the oil into a tablespoon of water, rub into your gums and leave overnight. Brush your teeth and rinse as normal in the morning.

570 BE FUSSY ABOUT FLUORIDE

Toothpaste containing fluoride is a wise investment. Fluoride kills bacteria and is also assimilated into the teeth, strengthening them and making them more resistant to decay.

571 RASPBERRY REMOVER

Rub crushed raspberries onto your teeth. The antioxidants and fruit acid will remove stains and leave your teeth looking really white. Rinse well afterwards.

572 SMOKE-FREE SMILE

Nicotine and tar in cigarettes stain your teeth, making them yellow in no time at all. Quit smoking and you'll have whiter teeth and more spare cash to spend on pampering treats.

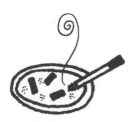

573 BANISH NAIL BITING

Chewing your nails can wreck your teeth, especially if the enamel is already weakened from consuming fizzy drinks (soda) and sweets (candy). Over time, a nail-biting habit can lead to trips to the dentist as well as salon visits – two reasons to quit now.

574 SIP WITH A STRAW

If you must drink dark-coloured drinks like coffee, tea or cola, always use a straw. It prevents the drink from swishing around in your mouth and staining your teeth.

575 CONTRAST CONTROL

You can make your teeth look instantly brighter without expensive whitening treatment by applying fake tan or bronzer to your face!

576 LIP SERVICE

For a quick whitening boost use a blue-toned, glossy red lipstick. Avoid orange and yellow tones as they can make teeth look yellow. Pale, frosted shades tend to make your teeth look dull as do matte finishes.

577 SALTY SMILE

Great lightening results can be seen if you brush your teeth with a combination of mustard oil and salt. It's much cheaper than a home-whitening kit.

578 MINTY FRESH

Why pay for a breath freshener that will give you minty breath when fresh mint is easy to grow yourself? Make your own mouth spray by pouring boiling water over fresh mint leaves and leaving overnight. Decant into a sterilized spray bottle and add a tablespoon of vodka to preserve. Store in the refrigerator.

579 UNPAID PROTECTION

If you're going to be drinking red wine or coffee, protect your teeth by coating them with a thin layer of petroleum jelly. The coating acts as a cheap but clever barrier to prevent staining.

580 RINSE AND SHINE

Stir a teaspoon of white apple cider vinegar into a glass of water to make an effective teeth-whitening rinse.

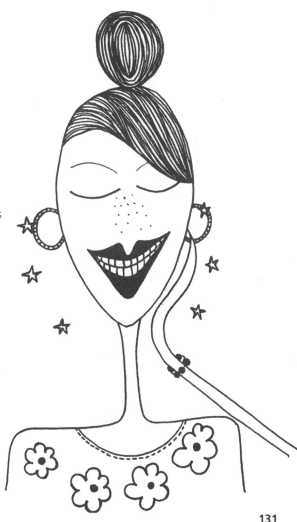

581 CHEW BETWEEN BRUSHES

Saliva is a powerful cleaner. Chewing sugar-free gum stimulates saliva and cleans your teeth, which is especially good after a meal if you aren't able to brush your teeth.

582 AVOCADO BREATH

If the root of your bad breath is acid indigestion, a cheap and easy solution is to eat some avocado. This healthy fruit effectively boosts digestion, preventing food from sitting in your stomach for too long.

583 PEARLY APPEAL

Apples contain pectin, which can help to neutralize food odours. So the next time you have a spicy curry or garlicky dinner, have an apple for dessert.

584 BREATH OF SUNSHINE

Eat a handful of sunflower seeds and drink a glass of water to treat bad breath. This low-calorie snack doesn't contain sugar or foul-tasting sweetener unlike many store-bought breath-freshener mints.

fragrances

585 STRIKE OIL

You can get perfume oils from health-food stores that smell exactly like some branded perfumes but cost a lot less. They tend to last much longer as well, due to the absence of alcohol.

586 DON'T GET SUCKED IN

Advertising suggests you can buy the glamour of a celebrity by dabbing on scent that has their name on the box, but you can often find similar-smelling fragrances for half the price. Take a sample of the star's perfume and compare it with cheaper ones to find a match.

587 RUSH FOR REFILLS

If your signature scent is expensive, ask at the beauty counter if they do refills. Many brands offer a refillable bottle – cheaper than splurging on the expensive packaging each time you run out.

588 SEARCH THE STORES

Different stores sell exactly the same branded bottle of perfume at different prices. And some may have special offers on your favourite, so always shop around to make savings.

589 JANUARY SALES

Stores bulk-buy perfumes before Christmas and so often have a surplus to get rid of in January. This is the best time to look for two-for-one and half-price offers. Other great dates are just after Valentine's Day or Mother's Day.

590 BE YOUR OWN PERFUMIER

Stir four to eight drops of your favourite essential oil into a little vodka. Leave for two days, then stir in 2 tablespoons of distilled water. Let it sit another couple of days before using it. The perfume can be stored in a dark-coloured glass bottle for six months.

591 PROLONG YOUR PERFUME

To help your favourite perfume retain its scent for longer, keep it away from damaging sunlight. Place it in its original box and store in a cool, dark place, such as a drawer.

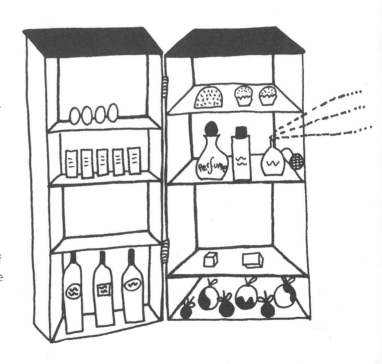

592 BOUQUET OF ROSES

Make your own sweetly scented rose oil fragrance. Place three handfuls of dried rose petals into a glass jar with a screw-top lid. Pour in almond oil to within about 12 mm (½ in) of the brim. Put the jar in a pan of simmering water and leave in the water until the oil has removed all of the colour from the petals. Strain and decant in a lidded, dark glass container. Store for six months in a cool, dark place.

593 EAU DE TOILETTE OR EAU DE PARFUM?

The bottle that represents better value depends on your spraying style. Eau de parfum is more concentrated, and therefore expensive, which is perfect if you just dab a little here and there. But if you like to spritz your perfume all over, then eau de toilette will last longer.

594 SCENTS AND SENSIBILITY

Don't wait until your favourite scent is all gone. When you start running low, find out if any friends or family are planning a trip abroad and ask them to get you some duty free. You'll often find that male friends have no plans to use their perfume allowance.

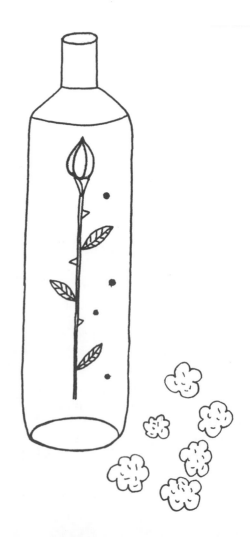

595 GIVE PERFUME A PULSE

Apply perfume in dabs to pulse points working from the toes up. These warm spots accentuate the smell, so a little will go a long way. Dab your ankles, behind your knees, your throat, wrists and the crooks of each elbow.

596 SIGNATURE SCENT

Studies show that men have more powerful memories of women who have a signature smell, so kick your addiction to bottle buying and stick to the one perfume that suits you, day and night. You will become more memorable (and better off!) instantly.

597 SCENT OF THE ORIENT

Some perfumes are very 'heavy', while others are 'light' and perfect for a sunny day. But if you choose a scent carefully, you can find one bottle that will be suitable for any time of day and whatever the weather. Oriental, also known as amber, scents tend to last longer and have the complex spicy notes needed to remain interesting.

598 THROW A PERFUME PARTY

We all have perfectly good perfumes that we're bored with. Instead of buying a new bottle, arrange for a few friends to gather up their unloved fragrances and host a perfume party.

599 HEAVEN-SCENT SOAK

Down to your last few drops of perfume? Mix it with baby oil and add to your bath for a soak that will leave your skin soft and beautifully scented.

600 AS MUCH AS YOU CAN CARRY!

Perfume is usually a lot cheaper at the airport, so check out the rules and regulations on how much you are allowed to buy, then stock up.

601 HAVE A NOSE ON THE NET

The internet is usually the cheapest place to buy perfume as web-based companies don't have to cover the cost of store overheads in their prices. Just make sure it's a reputable site and that you're not buying a fake.

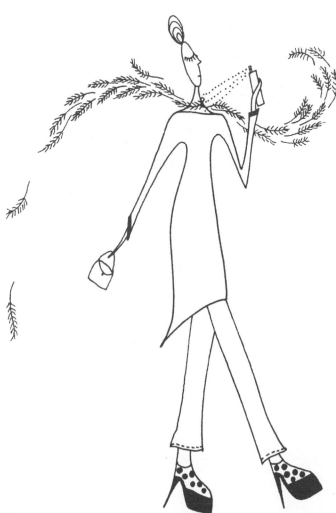

602 SINGLE LAYERS ONLY

Perfume brands encourage you to buy their full range of scented products including soap, shower gel and deodorant, by claiming that these extra items help layer the scent. However, provided you choose long-lasting perfume, it's fine to use cheap, unscented basics elsewhere.

603 BOTTLE COLLECTING

When you've used all of your special perfume, don't throw the bottle away. If it's a special-edition bottle (such as one produced for Christmas) it could become a collectors' item. Even within the first year some bottles have been known to increase by ten times in value.

604 DON'T BE A FOLLOWER

Love your friend's perfume? Don't rush out and buy it. Perfume reacts differently with an individual's skin, so it may not smell the same on you. Be sure to try her scent on your skin before making any rash and costly decisions.

605 DON'T DO DEPARTMENT STORES

Big stores are the prime destinations for perfume buyers, so they keep prices high. Try the supermarkets instead, who tend to be much more competitive with pricing.

606 MISTRUST MISTS

Body sprays and mists don't last long. Their fragrance fades quickly so you'll have to keep refreshing it all day. Choose more concentrated perfumes that last longer and you won't have to apply them so often.

607 MAXIMIZING MOISTURE

Perfume evaporates quickly on dry skin, so make sure you moisturize (using an economical and unscented moisturizer) before spraying on your perfume. Your scent will last all day and you'll find the bottles last much longer.

608 STICK YOUR SCENT TO YOU

Make your perfume really go the distance by applying a little petroleum jelly to the points on your body on which you plan to spray, particularly if you have oily skin. The perfume will cling to the jelly and the scent will linger for hours.

do-it-yourself body treatments

609 TAKE YOUR CUE

This scrub will combat dry skin and soothe sore areas. Mix one peeled and grated cucumber with a little milk and sugar to make a thin paste. Leave for five minutes to let the ingredients combine and then scrub over your body, concentrating on elbows, knees and ankles. Rinse off.

610 CREAM-FREE CURE

Massage boosts blood flow and aids the removal of toxins and fluids. You should gently knead cellulite areas, working in a motion towards your heart. Then use your knuckles to massage in the same direction.

611 SENSITIVE SCRUB

If you have dry or sensitive skin, try this gentle recipe. Mix a handful of oatmeal with a tablespoon of almond oil for a soothing, moisturizing scrub.

612 INVEST IN MITTS

Instead of wasting money on body scrubs that end up down the plughole, invest in a pair of exfoliation mitts and use them to lather up body wash for a daily all-over exhilarating clean. They'll last for years.

613 DAB AWAY DRYNESS

If you suffer from dry skin on your body, don't overmoisturize as this can actually exacerbate the problem. Instead, apply a thin layer of gentle body lotion straight after bathing or showering.

614 GIVE CREAM THE BRUSH-OFF

Stop buying expensive cellulite creams – there's absolutely no proof they work. Instead, buy a body brush and gently dry-brush your skin every day. This will improve your circulation and lymphatic drainage, which can improve stubborn cellulite.

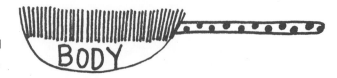

615 TONE UP WITH TURMERIC

This invigorating spice makes a great cellulite-busting body paste. Mix 1 heaped tablespoon of flour with 1 teaspoon of turmeric and a little milk or natural (plain) yogurt. Brush onto your skin using circular movements, then rinse well to avoid staining your towels.

616 NICE AND SPICY

This invigorating scrub improves circulation. Stir together 150 g (1¾ US cups) of flour, 2 tablespoons each of ground mustard and crushed coriander seeds, 200 ml (¾ US cup) of orange juice and 100 ml (½ US cup) of water. Work over your body and then rinse with warm water.

617 EASE THE PAIN

This scrub stimulates the circulation and will soothe muscular aches and pains after a hard day or exercise. Mix 2 tablespoons ground coffee beans with 1 teaspoon of cinnamon and 1 teaspoon of freshly chopped ginger. Gently rub over sore muscle areas as you shower.

618 SOAK IN A CUP

Lots of skincare products that claim to restore the skin's natural glow contain green tea. You can achieve the same without the hefty price tag by simply dropping a couple of green tea bags into your bath water.

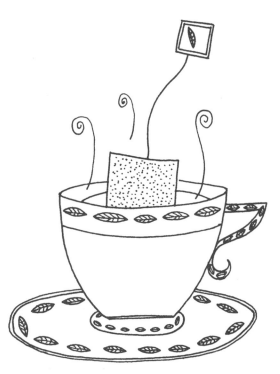

618 ORANGES AND LEMONS

For an invigorating morning wake-up call, squeeze the juice and pulp of one orange and one lemon into a bowl and mix in 4 tablespoons of oatmeal to make a paste. Rub onto clean skin then rinse off.

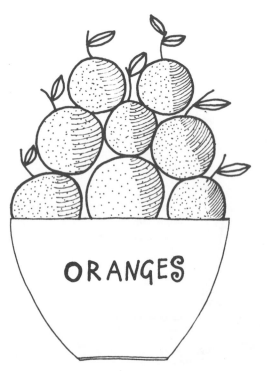

ORANGES

620 GO BANANAS

This recipe makes a moisturizing body mask for dry skin. Put a banana in a blender and blend until soft. Mix in 200 g (scant 1 US cup) of natural (plain) yogurt and about 130 g (generous ½ US cup) of butter. Chill in the refrigerator. Massage the mixture into your skin, leave it on for 20 minutes, then have a nice warm bath to rinse it off.

621 GOOD ENOUGH TO EAT!

Mix together a tablespoon each of honey, cocoa and salt. Gently massage this mix all over your body. The salt exfoliates, the honey provides a moisturizing effect, while antioxidant-rich cocoa is thought to help fight premature ageing.

622 STRETCH MARK SOLUTION

There's no need to save up for expensive laser treatment to fade stretch marks. You can speed up the skin's natural healing process by rubbing in vitamin E oil or aloe vera gel every day. Repeat religiously and they'll start to fade in weeks.

623 ESSENTIAL EXTRAS

A few drops of essential oil added to unscented body lotion and massaged daily into problem areas can work wonders. Juniper decreases excessive fluids, grapefruit helps remove toxins, rosemary tones and geranium boosts circulation.

624 TIME FOR TEA

This scrub is for exfoliating delicate areas such as your neck and chest. Mix 2 tablespoons of green tea leaves with 1 tablespoon of uncooked brown rice, 1 teaspoon honey and enough almond oil to make a paste. Rinse well.

625 BATH OF OATS

Buy a bag of cheap oats at the supermarket and wrap a handful in a tea towel. Tie the top with string and hang from your bath tap (faucet). Let the water run through the oats to create a creamy soak that will soften your skin. The oat bag can then be used as a cloth to wash your skin.

626 KIWI FRUIT REVITALIZER

Kiwi is known for its fruit acids and cleansing properties, and it is good for all skin types. Fruit acids help dissolve dead skin cells, so this kiwi scrub will remove dull flaky skin, revealing softer, fresher skin. Blend two kiwi fruits with a handful of salt and 2 tablespoons of honey – then scrub away. Rinse well to finish.

627 SELF-SERVICE SPRAY TAN

Why strip off in front of strangers at the beauty salon when you can get a bottle of spray tan from the store for a fraction of the price? Spray applicators make it easy to get an even tan, even on those hard-to-reach places.

628 GLOW ON

Prolong your golden glow, and cut back on expensive tanning products, by exfoliating and moisturizing your skin before you apply spray tan. Believe it or not, if you exfoliate every other day you will actually maintain an even, bronzed look for longer.

629 CLARIFYING CLEANSE

Instead of bubble bath, mix four parts cheap red wine with one part honey and add to running water. This combination will detoxify and moisten your skin.

630 SOFTENING BODY OIL

To make your own post-shower body oil, mix two parts almond oil with one part jojoba or sesame oil. Apply while your skin is still moist for maximum benefits.

631 STREAK-FREE FINISH

If you are applying fake tan after a shower or bath, always give the room a chance to air. Being in a hot, steamy room will make your skin perspire, giving your tan a streaky finish and making a second coat necessary.

632 CELLULITE-BUSTING COFFEE

Coffee is one of the main ingredients found in many cellulite creams. So rather than paying out huge sums on miracle creams, just add a shot of espresso to your normal body lotion for the same stimulating effect.

lifestyle tricks

633 GO SMOKE-FREE

There's no point spending money on fancy moisturizers if you still smoke the odd cigarette or allow people to smoke around you. Unless your skin is in a smoke-free zone it will lose elasticity and be unable to hold moisture.

634 GET MORE ZZZZS

Sleep is when we regain energy and rebuild our tissues and cells. So a free and instant way to give your face a lift and revitalize your skin is to make sure you're getting enough of it. Sleep will help to banish dark circles under your eyes and lift your mood.

635 CHANGE YOUR SLEEP POSITION

Curling up on your side in the foetal position can create wrinkles and creases around the eyes where skin is thinnest. Train yourself to sleep on your back at night and you'll wake up with smoother skin.

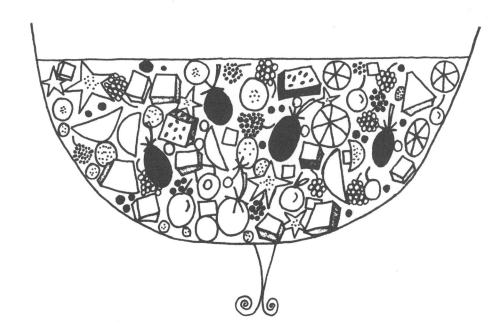

636 DITCH JUNK FOOD

Eating processed foods and ready-meals all the time will stop your skin and hair getting the nutrition they need to look great. Eat more fresh fruits and vegetables, wholegrains and fish, and you'll glow and shine without the need for expensive products.

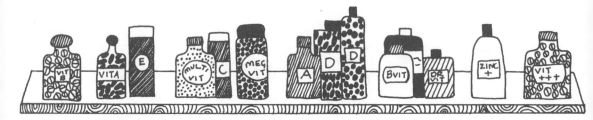

637 MIRACLE PILLS

If you are really worried about wrinkles, investing in a good multivitamin (as well as eating a healthy diet with plenty of fruit and veg) will save you money on expensive creams by ensuring you're not missing out on any vital anti-ageing nutrients.

638 DRINK LESS BOOZE

Saying bye-bye to booze will save you money instantly and your skin and body will thank you for it. Alcohol dehydrates you, making your face dull and dry, and drinking to excess is also likely to give you dark shadows under your eyes.

639 GET MOVING

Physical activity doesn't just make your body look better; it boosts your circulation, so ensuring that your skin gets all the nutrients it needs to stay soft. It also supplies your hair follicles with oxygen and the other goodies they require to keep your locks shiny and full of bounce.

640 DITCH THE COFFEE

Although coffee gives you a fast pick-me-up, too much caffeine can stop your body absorbing nutrients and dehydrate you, leaving skin lacklustre and triggering the appearance of dark circles.

641 FRUITY START

While you sleep your body is detoxifying, which is very important for healthy skin. Eating a heavy breakfast forces your body to stop this cleansing process and to start digesting food. A good idea is to choose fresh, ripe fruits for your first meal of the day – they require very little digestion and so will give your body a few more hours to finish the repair work.

642 MORE ME-TIME

Too many women don't take time out for themselves and end up feeling overloaded and frazzled. Pleasure is a nutrient in itself, so even if it's just 10 minutes a day, set aside time just to relax, read, whatever you like to do. You'll feel happier and less stressed, and it will show in your appearance.

643 EAT BETTER FAT

Revise your diet to replace saturated fats with healthy ones, such as the omega-3 fatty acids found in oily fish. Good fats regulate hormones and plump up the skin by keeping cell walls hydrated and flexible.

644 LOSE WEIGHT, AGE SLOWER

According to some experts, obesity accelerates the ageing process even faster than smoking. Obesity creates a constant state of heightened oxidative stress (free radical activity) that damages skin and causes wrinkles. Another good reason to shed those extra pounds!

645 SEE SOME DAYLIGHT

In the winter many of us suffer from low levels of vitamin D – produced when sunlight hits bare skin – which can leave us tired, pale and feeling low. Try to get at least 20 minutes of sunshine a day in the winter and early spring months by taking a brisk lunchtime walk.

646 THE SWEET TRUTH

When broken down by the body sugar sticks to collagen – the protein that keeps skin elastic – making it stiff and inflexible. The result? Wrinkles. So stay clear of sweet processed foods as much as possible and choose natural fruit sugars and honey instead.

647 AND RELAX...

When you're under pressure your adrenal glands release cortisol, a stress hormone that can damage skin and make you crave fatty food, along with other negative health consequences. Exercise regulates cortisol, but so can listening to music, meditation and breathing exercises.

648 GO NUTS

If you must snack between meals then give your skin a quick boost by munching on antioxidant-rich unsalted nuts. Pumpkin seeds, raisins, carrots, dried blueberries or cranberries, and fresh cherries are also good alternative snacks.

649 STRIKE A POSE

As well as reducing stress, yoga supports endocrine function and improves circulation. Inversion poses such as shoulder stands or headstands are also good for massaging the thyroid gland and relieving held-in stress in areas such as clenched jaws furrowed brows – prime wrinkle spots.

650 START INSIDE OUT

Dealing with beauty problems when they appear on the surface is much more expensive than developing a complete regime that helps protect your skin and boost your hair from the inside out. Good diet and skincare hygiene are therefore your most effective prevention tools.

651 CHEW LIKE A LADY

Chewing food carefully and completely is not only important for your maintaining a healthy weight. Failure to break down food properly can lead to the production of excess toxins, which leads to a bloated tummy and puffy eye bags.

652 AVOID BRIGHT LIGHTS

Research proves that basking under bright indoor lighting all day every day can cause pigment changes in the skin, including melasma (dark patches on the face). So, if you work in an office try to position yourself away from overhead lights – or consider applying sunscreen.

cost-free confidence tricks

653 FORM A LASTING IMPRESSION
Remember that after the first ten seconds, most people won't judge you on the way you look. If your inner beauty shines through you will make a good impression and people will respond positively to you.

654 MAKE LIKE A MOVIE STAR
Like anything else, beauty needs to be 'sold'. Try deliberately looking and acting more confident. If you add extra zing to the way you come across, people will respond to you more positively – and that in turn will make you feel even better about yourself.

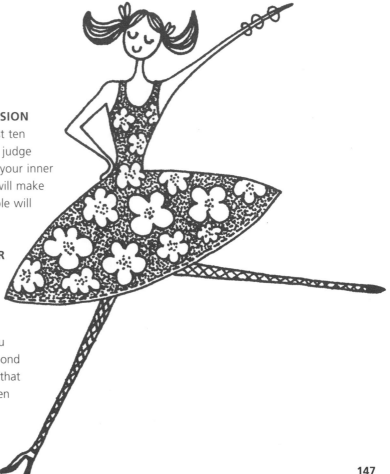

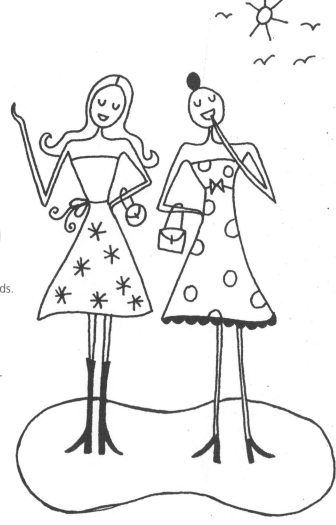

655 RECRUIT SOME BOOSTERS

Instead of filling your bathroom with expensive beauty treatments, surround yourself with some different confidence boosters – your friends. If you spend time with people who tell you how beautiful you are, you will soon feel – and see – the positive effects.

656 BREATHE LIKE A BABY

This quick meditation technique can produce a remarkable calming effect if you experience a sudden pang of low self-confidence. Lie on the floor, be quiet and place your hands on your stomach. Breathe from your stomach, letting it rise and fall like a pair of bellows.

657 FAKE IT

Just as applying your favourite lipstick can make a difference to your mood, the first step to feeling better about yourself is often to start acting confidently, even if you're feeling down. Act like you feel beautiful and people will respond to that self-confidence.

658 IGNORE THE COMPETITION

Nothing ruins a beautiful face like a frown, so don't make comparisons that will only make you miserable. In particular, don't compare yourself with the celebrities you see in the magazines – their pics are airbrushed so what you see is not real!

659 MAKE A HEALTHY CHOICE

The health benefits of having a nutritious salad and a glass of water for lunch are not immediately apparent, but if you're feeling low the confidence-boosting effects can be beneficial. Feeling like you've given your body a healthy treat makes you feel instantly better about yourself, which is a great beauty pick-me-up.

660 SEIZE THE DAY

Make an effort to look good every day and you'll instantly feel more attractive. Give yourself enough time to blow-dry your hair, apply a touch of make-up and pick out your most stylish and brightly coloured clothes.

661 TAKE UP SPACE

Don't spend money on your make-up and clothes only to disappear into a corner at social functions. Allow yourself to take centre stage with broad gestures and a clear, definite voice tone.

662 FIVE-SECOND FIX

If you ever find yourself feeling bad about the way you look, use this quick strategy: remember a time when you felt really confident in your appearance, then take a deep breath and as you let it out, allow yourself to feel good.

663 STAND TALL

A confident posture costs nothing and is better than an expensive new outfit. Hold your head high and keep your shoulders back. Place your feet hip-width apart so that you're well balanced and maintain eye contact with the other person.

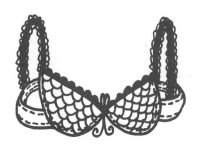

664 GIVE TO RECEIVE

Remember, the best way to get that beauty-enhancing confidence boost you require is to compliment others. Make an effort to tell people you meet or work with how great they look, especially when they've made an effort or look unhappy. That way people will think to return the compliment when you need it the most.

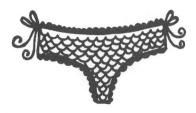

665 A SEXY SECRET

Underwear doesn't have to be seen by anyone else to be special. You can add a sexy swagger to your walk simply by wearing your favourite underwear under your work clothes.

666 ACCENTUATE THE POSITIVE

Too much make-up focuses on fixing the bits you don't like about your face. It's much more rewarding to find something you do like about your face – perhaps you have great bone structure or a rosebud mouth? Now concentrate on playing up these good bits.

667 TELL YOURSELF YOU'RE BEAUTIFUL

A self-compliment may sound cheesy, but there's no point spending lots of money on make-up if you don't believe you're worth it. The first step to being beautiful is feeling good about yourself, so get rid of the inner-critic and say something positive.

668 KEEP SMILING

A smile really is worth a million dollars. A positive expression will not only give the impression of confidence and make you feel better about yourself, it will make you approachable and people will respond well and want to talk to you.

668 TAKE A BREAK FROM YOURSELF

Role-play doesn't have to be limited to the bedroom – or require an audience. You can get a real beauty boost just by pretending to be someone else for a day. There's no need to tell anyone – just do your make-up differently, change your style of dress, maybe even wear a wig.

670 CHANGE IT UP

If you always play safe and stick to the same make-up routine, the positive effects will start to wear off after a while. There's no need to buy new make-up; just use what you've got a little differently – wear your eyeliner a little thicker or gloss your lips after applying lipstick.

671 GO NATURAL

Have the confidence to leave the house without any make-up on. It will reduce your dependence on too many products and save you money. Start with a trip to the supermarket.

complementary & holistic beauty

672 GIVE IT THE NEEDLE

If you have private acupuncture sessions to ease a bad back or migraines, you could save cash by visiting your GP. Talk your doctor through the problem and they may be able to refer you for acupuncture at a reduced rate; check that your insurance will cover it.

673 IT'S GOOD TO TALK

If you are looking for a holistic therapist, it's a good idea to ask for recommendations from friends. Smaller practices that tend to offer cheaper-priced treatments don't have money for advertising and so rely on word of mouth.

674 CHECK YOUR SOURCES

Local hairstylists are the best people to ask for a recommendation for great-priced complementary therapy treatment. They're a wonderful source of information as they pick up tips when chatting with clients.

675 FOLLOW YOUR NOSE

Aromatherapy candles and oils are always cheaper after Christmas so stock up in January. However, don't just buy any old aromatherapy candle. Research the right oil for you – relaxing, energizing or balancing – so that you don't waste money on products you'll never use.

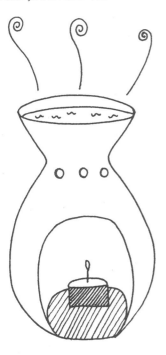

676 WINTER WARMER

A great Ayurvedic relaxation treatment for cold winter nights is a ginger-infused bath. Place 2–3 tablespoons of freshly grated ginger in a piece of muslin (cheesecloth), tie it to the bath tap (faucet) and run warm water over it. Alternatively, put 2 tablespoons of ginger powder straight into your bath water.

677 THE FINER POINTS

Reflexology may help you to unwind but professional sessions are pricey. However, this is one therapy you can actually do to yourself. See if your local library has a book on reflexology or research techniques on the internet. Get a friend involved and you can practise what you learn on each other.

678 LEFT TO LINGER

Essential oils can be damaged by direct light so only buy them in dark-coloured glass bottles and avoid those on display. Also avoid plastic bottles and rubber stoppers, because the oils will dissolve the plastic, become contaminated and lose their potency.

679 CARING CALENDULA

If you suffer from dry, chapped skin, pick up a tube of calendula cream from your local health store. Apply a small amount and this natural plant-based cream should clear the problem in no time. A little goes a long way so a small tube will last you longer than a tub of expensive moisturizer.

680 A TASTE OF THE ORIENT

Beauty salons and spas charge a lot for relaxing herbal therapies but you can often get the same treatments at far lower prices from Chinese medical centres. Most towns have one these days, so check local listings. Don't be afraid to try something different; you could make some big savings.

681 INDIAN BEAUTY

Invest in neem oil, the basis of most Ayurvedic beauty treatments. It's known as liquid gold because it's meant to have purifying and healing properties. You can get a big bottle for next to nothing in most health-food stores. Add to bath water or use it as a massage oil.

682 SENSIBLE SCENT SHOPPING

Avoid buying aromatherapy products from cosmetics stores because they usually sell impure oils, adulterated with cheaper chemical ingredients. Herbalists and health-food stores are the best places to buy essential oils as you'll be paying for quality.

683 HOLISTIC CELLULITE HELP

To achieve the same effect as a salon hydrotherapy jet treatment, direct a cold shower head at your ankle and very slowly up the back of your leg. Then do the same with hot water. Repeat a couple of times and finish with cool water. This boosts circulation, leaving skin looking firmer and less pitted.

684 CHEST BATH

When you've got a cold, try this Ayurvedic remedy. Mix 50 ml (1/4 US cup) sesame oil, a 2–3 drops of ginger and cedarwood essential oils, 1 teaspoon of tamarind spice powder and a crushed garlic clove. Warm the paste gently and rub it onto your chest. Leave for 40 minutes to help clear your chest; also use it as a soothing rub for aches and pains.

do-it-yourself massages

685 FACE SOOTHER

To give yourself a face massage, start by working your fingertips in small circles, moving steadily down from your forehead, around your temples and over your cheeks. Then work your fingers along each side of your nose, and along your jaw, making sure you don't pull downwards on your skin.

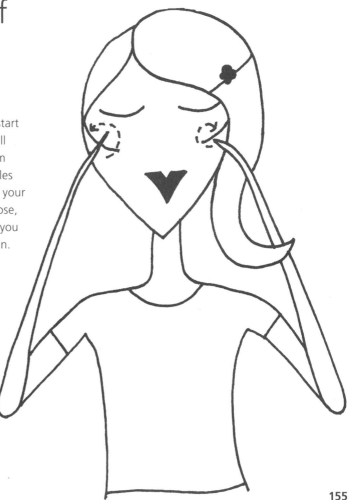

686 ENERGY BOOSTER

Rub your back just above your kidneys –
at waist level where the tissue is still soft.
Rub briskly with your fists in a circular
motion. This should leave you feeling
energized as it's a key invigorating area
in traditional Chinese medicine.

687 KEEP IT SIMPLE

Don't splash out on expensive massage
bars or oils; a moderate amount of ordinary
hand or body cream will work just as well –
and you won't be left with greasy skin.

688 GET WARMED UP

Relaxing tense muscles
with a hot bath or
shower before a
massage will make
the treatment twice as
effective. This advice
applies whether you're
massaging yourself,
your partner is obliging
you with one, or you're
going to a salon.

689 CALF CONTROL

Sit in a chair and place your feet flat on the
floor. Starting at your ankle, press the sides
of your index fingers against the back of
your calf and move your hands up to your
knee. Use your hands to wiggle the calf
muscle. Then using circular motions gently
press your fist into the calf muscle. Repeat
on the other leg.

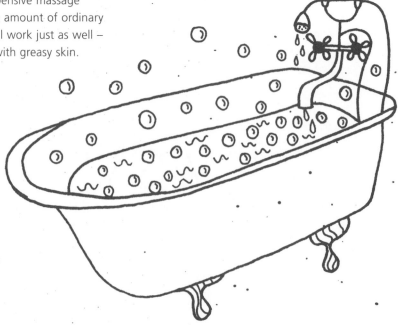

690 THIGH HIGH

Keeping your hands flat and using them alternately, stroke from knee to hip, around the thigh. Next squeeze your muscle between your thumb and fingers and then let go, working your way from your knee upwards in a straight line. Start with the front of your thigh and move onto the back and sides.

691 BRACING BACK RUB

To target your lower back, lace your fingers and place them on your lower back between your lower ribcage and your hipbone, and slowly rock your hands back and forth. Next, form a loose fist and using the back of your knuckles push into the same area a little harder.

692 MIX YOUR OILS

Massage oil is extremely easy to make at home. Just mix a couple of drops of essential oil with 50 ml (¼ US cup) of a base oil, such as almond or olive oil. Try adding lemon or orange essential oils for a refreshing scent.

683 POST-WORKOUT PUMMEL

This works on any muscle you can reach. Place your palm over the sore muscle, keep your fingers together and form a 'V' with your thumb and index finger. Glide your hand up and down the muscle, applying just enough pressure to indent your skin.

684 HEALING HEAD HELP

For a soothing head massage that relieves stress and stiffness, work your fingers and thumbs in circular motions over your scalp. Start the top of your neck and behind your ears and work your way up over your crown to your temples, working right and left simultaneously. Rub any tender areas extra firmly.

685 NAIL NECK PAIN

Place your left hand on your right shoulder and your right hand on your left shoulder. Tilt your head to one side and press down with your fingertips one at a time. Press down on any areas that are sore until the pain subsides. Tilt your head in the opposite direction and repeat.

696 SOOTHE A TIRED BODY

Rub the length of the outside of your thighs and arms, buttocks and stomach vigorously with a little almond, juniper and cypress essential oils, combined in equal amounts. As well as easing aches, these oils are also great for targeting cellulite.

697 PLAY SOLO FOOTSIE

Apply pressure to the sole of your foot with your thumbs and knuckles, working from your heel towards your toes. Next hold each toe firmly and move it from side to side. Finally roll your thumbs between the bones of the ball of your foot. Repeat on the other foot.

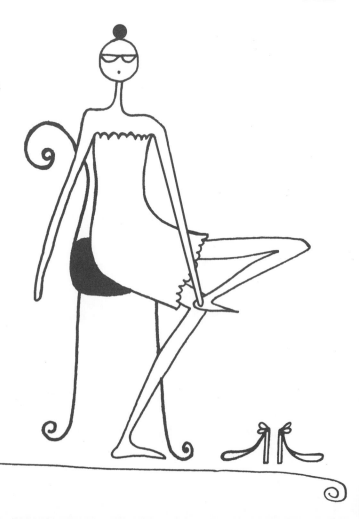

massages for your partner or friends

688 FACE IT

Use your middle fingers to stroke upwards from the chin and then from the centre of the nose outwards to the sides of the face – as if painting on cat whiskers. Next, work upwards across the forehead. Massage the face in the same direction using circular strokes. Avoid massaging downwards and in the eye areas.

689 HEAVENLY HEAD RUB

Massage the temples by moving your thumbs in small circles, then slide the tips of your index and middle fingers to the ends of the eyebrows by the nose, pressing in a circular motion. Next, walk your fingers up from the outer ends of the eyebrows to the scalp. Finish by massaging the head as if you were shampooing the hair.

700 DIFFERENT STROKES

As the masseuse, start slowly and gently and learn your partner's likes and dislikes when it comes to firmness. Start with long, gliding strokes from the lower back, up towards the neck and back down again.

701 VARIETY IS THE SPICE OF LIFE

As well as depth, try alternating the speed of your movements when you massage. Going from slow, fingertip caresses to quick strokes is incredibly soothing.

702 BLADE RUNNER

Knead the muscles at the base of the neck. Then place your fingers pointing down, where the base of your partner's skull meets their neck, and knead gently. Finally, press down with the heel of your hand between their shoulder blades and spine.

703 ANYONE FOR TENNIS?

For an effective pressure reliever, put two tennis balls in a sock and place them under any tender spot along your back or hips while sitting on the sofa or lying down.

704 DO THE LEG WORK

Use your palms to rub the back of their thigh with long, upward strokes. Then place the heel of your hand on the bottom of the thigh muscle, above the knee, and firmly but gently slide it up the length of the thigh. Lastly, work the front of the thigh with long, upward palm strokes. Repeat on other leg.

705 TOOLS OF THE TRADE

Many household items can be used as massagers, but stick to soft, rounded items and avoid anything pointy. Golf balls are great for the soles of your feet, and a rolling pin is perfect for legs and arms.

706 BACK IT UP

Starting on their lower back, glide your hands up either side of the spine, over the shoulders and down the sides. Make a 'V' between your thumb and index finger and glide firmly up the back. Move your thumbs in small circles to work out any aches.

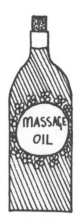

707 FAB FOOT RUB

Place both hands around the foot with your fingers on the sole and your thumbs on top. Move your thumbs between the tendons smoothly and firmly from the ankle towards the toes. Use enough pressure so that it's not ticklish, but not so much that it's painful. Next massage the sole of the foot, from the toes to the heel, by moving your thumbs in circular motions. Repeat on the other foot.

708 A GOOD SQUEEZE

Have your subject lie down on their back with one leg bent (foot flat on the floor, knee pointing up). Hold the knee stable so they can relax the bent leg. With your other hand, grab the back of the calf muscle and start squeezing and releasing all the way from the back of the knee down to the ankle.

709 SOCK IT TO 'EM

Pour uncooked rice into a sock. Tie a knot in it and place it in the microwave for one minute. When the rice is heated up, you can use the sock as a warm massager for use on sore areas.

710 HOT STONES

Collect flat, smooth stones in a variety of sizes. Wash them and put them in a casserole dish filled with water. Heat slowly in an oven set at a low temperature until they're warm, not boiling. Checking the temperature, place along the back for instant relief of muscle tension.

better-value treatments

711 CHIP AWAY THE COST

Chipping a recent manicure or pedicure is irritating. But don't worry – most nail salons offer a touch-up service that's cheaper than a full treatment. Go to your salon, taking the nail polish you used, and they'll make your nails look good as new in minutes.

712 FRIENDLY FREEBIES

Spas often have a 'take a friend for free' deal. Find yourself a partner in crime and you can grab great deals by splitting the cost. You may have to share a room, though, so make sure it's someone you get along well with!

713 LAST-MINUTE DEALS

Many hotels have a spa facility. They might not be as large as a dedicated spa, but if you just fancy lounging around in a pool and maybe having a facial, then you can save money by searching for a hotel with a spa on a last-minute travel website.

714 PRACTICE MAKES PERFECT

Beauty therapists learn their trade at beauty colleges. So if you fancy a cheap massage or beauty treatment, and you're willing to forego some of the trimmings, then find out whether your local college offers treatments by trainees.

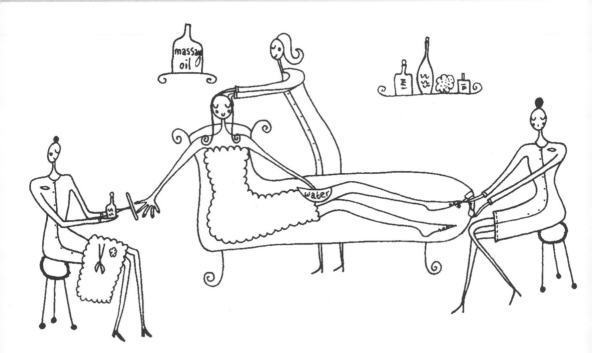

715 MIDWEEK MONEY SAVING

People usually visit at the weekend, so spas nearly always have weekday spaces to fill. Ask if they offer discounted prices for midweek stays. You're bound to find a cheaper deal if you're flexible on which nights of the week you visit.

716 HOST A PAMPERING PARTY

Invite over a group of mates who all want a beauty treatment. If you tell a local home-visit beauty therapist that you will have 10 to 20 customers for them, you'll be able to negotiate a discounted rate. Aim for 20 per cent off per person.

717 TREAT YOURSELF

Facials can be expensive, but there's a sneaky way to get more for your money. Beauty counters in department stores will often offer a free mini-facial if you buy at least two products from their range.

718 PHONE A FRIEND

Beauty therapists are always on the lookout for new clients, and will often show their appreciation with a free treatment if you refer a friend to them. Don't be afraid to ask.

719 LOYALTY CARD

Ask if your spa or salon offers rewards for loyalty. Many will give out cards on which you record your treatments and then after a certain number of visits you'll be rewarded with a free treatment.

720 BE IN THE KNOW

Always ask to be put on mailing lists for salons and cosmetic stores. You'll receive coupons and notices about upcoming specials and promotions, so you'll never miss a bargain.

create the perfect home spa

721 LIGHT DISPLAY

One of the techniques spas use to enhance relaxation is to employ clever lighting. Turn your bedroom into a post-bath relaxation zone by using a lava lamp or twinkling fairy (Christmas) lights.

722 WARMING WELCOME

There's nothing as luxurious as warmed towels. Ensure you enjoy the same toasty treat at home by hanging your towel and bathrobe on the radiator or giving them a spin in the tumble dryer before you step into the bath.

723 SCENT-SATIONAL SOAK

Grab a handful of lavender, oatmeal and rose petals, tie them up in a piece of muslin (cheesecloth) and hang it from the bath tap (faucet). The warm water will run through the bag, creating a soothing soak.

724 CHOCOLATE BLISS

Blend 150 g (1¾ US cups) of dried milk powder with 85 g (¾ US cup) of cocoa. Add the mixture to your bath for a luxurious treat. For a bubbly twist, mix in some bicarbonate of soda (baking soda).

725 KEEP YOUR MARBLES

Create a mini-foot massager by layering the bottom of a bowl with marbles before adding warm water. Run your feet over the marbles while they soak for a soothing massage.

726 TEATIME TREAT

For a cheap, healing herbal bath, throw a couple of peppermint or camomile tea bags into the running water and inhale deeply as you relax.

727 PUT BEAUTY ON ICE

A trick of the spa trade is to cool the skin after any firming or exfoliating treatment. Place an ice cube inside a small plastic bag and gently rub over your face for several minutes to plump and tone the skin.

728 SET THE SCENE

The whole point of a spa experience is to have some quality me-time, so make sure all of your commitments and responsibilities are taken care of. Turn off your mobile (cell) phone and unplug the home phone, put on some relaxing music and light some aromatic candles. Make sure no one will disturb you – and relax.

729 DRINK UP

Part of the spa detox experience involves upping your water intake, so for the same results at home keep a plastic jug of filtered water next to the bath, with a few slices of lemon in it. Alternate this with warm nettle tea to shift any toxins.

730 BLISSFUL BUBBLES

If your favourite part of a spa experience are the water massagers, you can recreate the effect by investing in a home bubble jet spa. These pump-powered cushioned mats stream bubbles and will cost you less than a single visit to a spa.

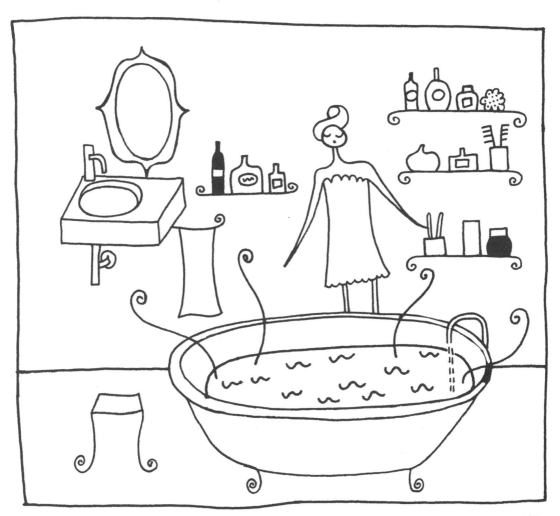

731 BERRY FINE BATH

This is an excellent way to combat dry skin. Blend 1½ tablespoons of castor oil with 150 ml (generous ½ US cup) of thick, natural (plain) yogurt, 200 g (1½ US cups) of blueberries and 750 ml (1½ US pints) of water until smooth and creamy. Pour half the mixture into running bath water and enjoy. Store the remaining in the fridge and use within 48 hours.

732 SPA-WORTHY SALT SCRUB

Mix 1 heaped tablespoon of sea salt with 12 drops of juniper essential oil. Add enough water to make a paste. Apply to damp skin in brisk circular strokes, concentrating on elbows, knees and feet, and rinse off. This scrub will exfoliate dead skin cells, cleanse the pores and eliminate toxins.

733 SOOTHING SALTS

To ease dry or sunburnt skin, mix a little aloe vera oil or gel with Epsom salts or sea salt. Add the mixture to lukewarm bath water.

734 SPRAY AWAY STRESS

Spa treatments often end with the therapist spritzing your face with a hydrating herbal mist. Create your own by making a cup of any flower or herbal relaxation-blend tea and add five drops each of lavender oil and basil oil. Cool and store in a sterilized spray bottle. Keep it on your desk at work and use it as a handy stress-buster.

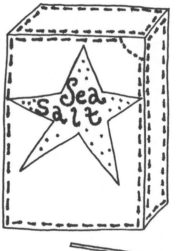

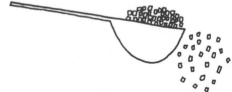

735 SEAWEED SLIMMER

A handful of fresh or dried seaweed added to warm bath water will help your body eliminate excess toxins. Sprinkle in with a few drops of rosemary essential oil to boost circulation and take the edge off the smell.

736 CRÈME BRÛLÉE

For cut-price real vanilla bath bubbles, blend together 200 ml (1 US cup) of almond oil, 100 ml of honey (scant ½ US cup), 100 ml (scant ½ US cup) of unperfumed liquid soap and 1 tablespoon vanilla extract. Pour into a plastic bottle and add about a quarter of the mix to warm bath water. Store in a cool, dark cupboard for up to three months.

737 MARVELLOUS MELTS

Melt 225 g (1 US cup) of cocoa butter, take it off the heat and stir in 225 g (8 oz) of bicarbonate of soda (baking soda), 75 g (scant ¾ US cup) of cornflour (cornstarch) and the juice of one lemon. Add a few drops of your favourite essential oil. Put into an ice-cube tray and freeze. Pop a couple into hot bath water for a moisturizing soak.

738 EXPLOSIVE FUN

To make fabulous bath bombs, put 200 g (7 oz) of bicarbonate of soda (baking soda) into a bowl, drizzle in 2 teaspoons of almond oil and the juice of one lemon and a 4 drops of an essential oil for fragrance. Hand-roll the mixture into balls approximately the size of golf balls and leave to dry on a sheet of greaseproof (waxed) paper until hard. Store in an airtight container for up to two weeks.

739 IT'S A WRAP

Stir 225 g (8 oz) of green clay, 2 heaped tablespoons of sea salt and 2 tablespoons of olive oil into a bowl of boiling water. Let the paste cool, but it should still be warm, and apply to your body. Wrap yourself in warm towels and sit and relax for 45 minutes. Take a shower – your skin should feel smoother and firmer and your silhouette should look a little slimmer.

buff body on a budget

740 DISCO DIVA

Just by dancing around your living room you can burn 100 calories in 15 minutes! So put on your favourite songs and boogie. Don't worry about looking or feeling silly, the more energetic your moves the better.

741 BASKET-CASE

At the supermarket, ditch the trolley (cart) in favour of a basket. By simply carrying your shopping you will tone your arm muscles and burn off as many calories as you would in a half-hour aerobics class.

742 BUTT BLASTER

This move will help you achieve a pert bottom. Stand at the bottom of the stairs, step onto the first step with your right foot, then your left, and then step down in the same order. Repeat 15 times, alternating your leading leg.

743 BURN IT IN THE BEDROOM

Sex lowers cholesterol and blood pressure, hones muscles and can burn as many calories as a short run. So grab your partner for a fun, free workout session.

744 DESK MOVES

Tone your inner thighs as you work by placing a water bottle between your knees while sitting up straight with your abs pulled in. Squeeze with your knees, release halfway and squeeze again. Repeat 16 times in a slow pulsing motion.

745 CALORIE-BURNING COMMUTE

Shape up while saving money on travel by walking to and from work. Brisk walking burns up to 400 calories an hour, is great for cardiovascular fitness and improves muscle tone.

746 BUSINESS BENEFITS

Many gyms offer discounts to employees of local businesses. Check with your employer, or ask at the gym and see if you can negotiate a good business deal.

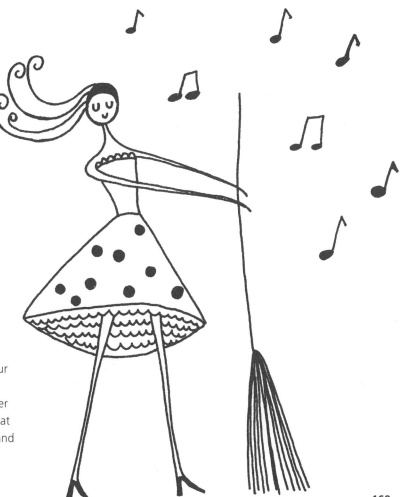

747 BE A HOUSE-PROUD HONEY

Forget the gym – housework can be a great body toner. Just mopping the floor for 30 minutes burns up to 200 calories. And you'll be left with a gleaming house instead of a pile of sweaty gym clothes.

748 IT'S A DOG'S LIFE

Investing in a furry friend can give you a better body. Walking the dog burns 360 calories an hour – for regular dog-walkers that's more than 2,500 per week! Plus walking is great for overall fat reduction and better muscle definition.

748 ESCALATOR EXERCISE

When taking an escalator don't just stand there. View the moving stairs as a chance for a quick free workout. Steps are great for shaping thighs and calves.

750 WEIGHTY DECISION

Work out at home rather than pay for an expensive gym. If you lack equipment, use cans of tomatoes or bottles of water for weights. Just make sure the weight in each hand is equal.

751 WHITTLE WHILE YOU WORK

This seated side stretch is a great way to trim your waist at your desk. With your arms raised over your head or on your hips, lean gently over to one side as far as you can safely and comfortably go. Repeat on the other side several times and whenever you have a spare moment.

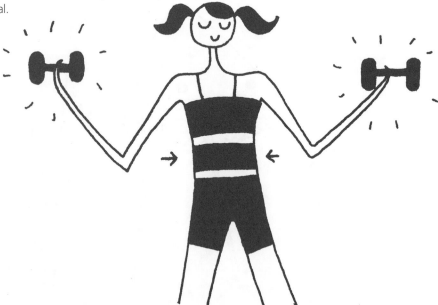

752 SIMPLE STEP CLASS

Why pay to do a step class when you have the perfect equipment at home? Walking up and down the stairs at a moderate pace burns up to 400 calories an hour and will quickly tone flabby thighs.

753 BARGAIN HUNTING

There's no need to break the bank when buying sports equipment. A search on a website selling second-hand goods will turn up plenty of cut-price gear. Charity (thrift) stores are also a haven for sports goods – especially just after Christmas.

754 BOARDROOM BUTT SQUEEZES

This great move will give you a pert behind and can be done while you're on the phone or typing up a report without anyone else noticing. Simply squeeze your buttock muscles in and hold for 30 seconds, then relax. Repeat 20 times.

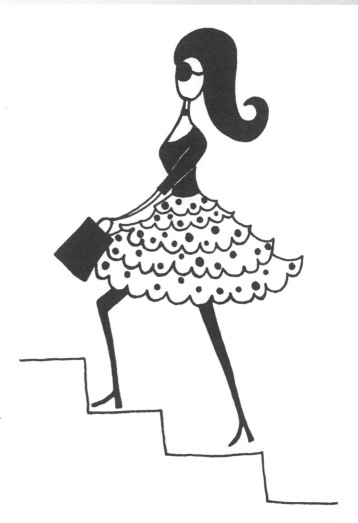

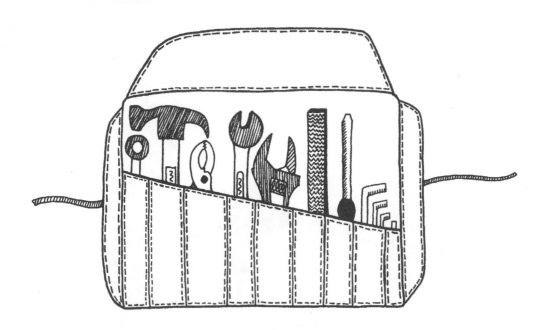

755 GET INTO DIY

Save money on decorators and gym membership by doing your own home maintenance. You'll tone your arms while painting walls and streamline your thighs as you squat to sand floors.

756 WORKOUT A BETTER DEAL

If your work hours are flexible, consider off-peak gym membership. Not only will your membership fees be cheaper but your workouts are likely to be quicker as you won't have to wait to use the equipment.

757 SET A BODY BENCHMARK

Turn a park bench into a gym bench by sitting down and gripping the edge either side of your hips. Ease yourself off the edge. Lift yourself up and down by bending your arms to a 90-degree angle. Repeat three sets of 15 for slim, sculpted arms.

758 LEARN TO HAGGLE

Make the most of current competition between local gyms. Call a few and ask what deal they can offer you, and don't be afraid to haggle or ask for a discount. The worst they can say is no, and you could end up saving loads.

759 TRY BEFORE YOU BUY

Lots of gyms offer free one-day or full-week passes so that you can give their services a trial run. So before signing up, give the facilities a try and decide whether you would really use them!

fake a facelift

760 WORK OUT WORRY

To minimize frown lines, rub your temples and forehead with your knuckles. Start from the centre of your forehead and move out towards the temples. Massage for two minutes to ease the appearance of wrinkles. This also relieves headaches.

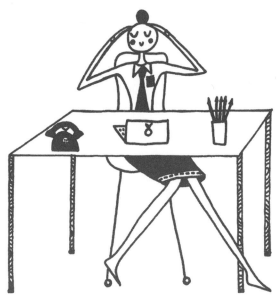

761 CREATE A YOUTHFUL GLOW

Apply cream pearl highlighter to your brow
bone, the top of your cheeks and the inner
corner of you eyes. This will lift your complexion,
making you look younger in the process.

762 KEEP AN EYE ON AGEING

Having perfectly groomed eyebrows helps
create the illusion of lifted lids. Plus, having
more skin showing between your brow bone
and eyelid opens up the entire eye area for
a more fresh-faced look.

763 INVEST FOR SUCCESS

Skip the expensive Botox and invest in a skin-
brightening face cream instead. These tighten
your skin and leave your complexion looking
radiant, knocking years off in the process.

764 BANISH BAGS

To fight discoloration and bags under
the eyes, rub your face gently on either
side of your nostrils. Gently rubbing
here releases the toxins that can
otherwise show up as blotches and
bags under your eyes.

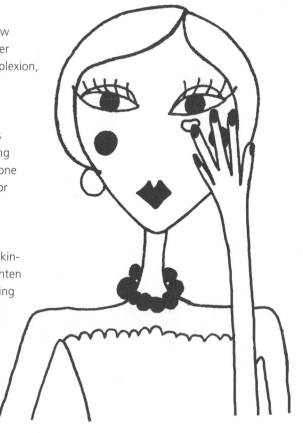

765 LIFT DROOPY EYES

Draw a line along your upper lashes with eyeliner, extending slightly further than the outer corner, and sloping upwards slightly. Line the bottom eyelid with a lighter shade to add to the lift effect.

766 CLEVER COMBING

To make the skin on your face look instantly tighter and lifted, try this much-used celebrity favourite. Pull your hair back as tightly as is comfortable from your face and secure in place with hairgrips (bobby pins).

767 YOUTHFUL PEEPERS

Cut out salty foods for at least three hours before bed. Salt triggers water retention, which can cause puffy eyes the next morning.

768 WIDE-AWAKE CLUB

Place three fingers under your eye and very gently pull down without closing your eyes. Hold for ten seconds and release. This will get the blood flowing to the skin under your eyes, which will help reduce puffiness.

769 FORGET TO FROWN

Stop worrying about laughter lines and smile! Over the years our faces lose fat and our brows lower, which makes your face look serious or cross in repose. But when you smile, your face lifts and your cheeks become rounder and more youthful. Smiling is the most natural facelift you can get.

770 LOSE YOUR LINES

To tone your cheeks and lessen the appearance of lateral lines, inhale and hold the air in your mouth with your cheeks puffed out like a trumpet player. Hold for as long as you can before slowly exhaling through your nostrils. Repeat five times. This is also a good stress-buster.

771 NATURAL NIP AND TUCK

Hold the underside of your chin with an open palm. Tilt your head back until you feel your throat skin stretching. Intensify the stretch by bringing your lower lip up over the upper one. Hold for 20 seconds and repeat ten times every day.

fake chiselled cheeks

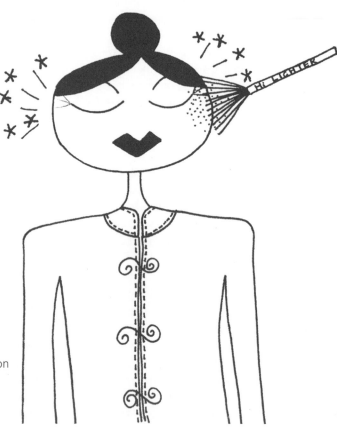

772 NATURALLY SCULPTED

For a more natural daytime look, apply a foundation that is a shade darker than your skin tone under your cheekbones instead of blusher. Apply highlighter to the top of your cheekbones to accentuate the look.

773 MAKE IT UP

Suck your cheeks in to find your natural cheekbones and then shade the area directly underneath with a bronze-toned blusher. Next, apply a paler pink or peach shade to the top of your cheekbone, creating the illusion of a more chiselled, slimmer face.

774 BOOSTING BOB

Angled bob haircuts, with sides that taper softly below the cheeks, can help create the illusion of higher, more angular cheekbones.

775 CHEEKY MOVES

Inhale and hold the air under your upper lip for a few seconds. Move it to your right cheek. Hold. Move the air to your left cheek. Hold. Move to your lower lip. Hold. Then blow out. This will firm up your cheeks and get them glowing.

776 GRIN AND BEAR IT

Push your chin out, and raise your bottom lip over your upper lip. Using your cheek muscles only, raise the corners of your mouth into a smile. Hold this position and count to five. Repeat three times a day for firmer cheeks.

fake a nose job

777 CREATE WIDER APPEAL

Apply a broad strip of highlighter or pale powder down the centre of your nose and blend well using a lighter foundation to enlarge a nose that's too thin.

778 THE PINOCCHIO EFFECT

Apply highlighter or pale powder over and under the tip of your nose. By drawing attention to the tip of your nose you will make it seem more prominent.

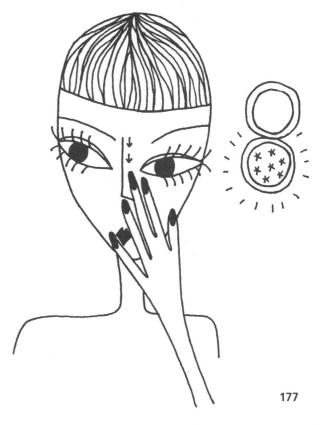

779 PERFECT POWDER

Highlights and shine tend to draw attention to features. However, matt powder applied to the nose will make it appear smaller.

780 DISTRACTION TECHNIQUES

If you dislike your nose, choose flamboyant, statement earrings to help distract attention away from the centre of the face. Go for studs, however, as very dangly earrings can accentuate a longer nose.

781 AVOID POINTING IT OUT

A centre parting is like an arrow pointing directly to your nose, so opt for a side parting instead. If your nose bends slightly to one side, part your hair on the opposite side to help balance it.

782 SLIM YOUR SNOUT

To create the illusion of a narrower nose, apply a matt bronzer down the sides of your nose. Then apply a thin stripe of pale powder highlighter down the bridge of your nose. Make sure to blend well to avoid a streaky finish.

783 DON'T BE BLUNT

Thick, blunt fringes (bangs) can look like a pelmet highlighting a larger nose. Softer, side-sweeping fringes are more flattering.

784 HAVE A RESTYLE

Talk to your hairstylist about styles that will best suit your face. Bear in mind that short, straight styles tend to emphasize the nose so opt for long, wavy locks instead.

785 GET SHORTY

To make a long nose seem shorter, blend a slightly darker foundation under your nose and up over the tip. Extend your blush application to just below the apples of your cheeks. This will make your cheeks appear to end lower down your face, putting things in proportion.

786 MIND THE BUMP

To hide a crooked nose, apply bronzer down the bridge of your nose stopping where the tip begins to protrude. Be sure to blend it well. A straight line of highlighter down the centre will also help make it look straighter.

fake lip-fillers

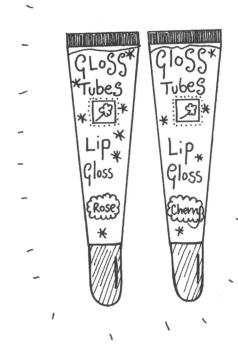

787 GLOSS OVER WEAKER POINTS

Make narrow lips appear fuller by applying a dab of gloss or a paler shade of lipstick in the centre of your lips to create the illusion of plumpness.

788 PENCIL IN YOUR POUT

Trace just outside your upper lip line using a slightly blunt lipliner. Fill in the new lip area with the pencil using very light pressure, so the outline still looks slightly darker. Then paint over the whole area with gloss.

789 PEARLY SMILE

Choose lipsticks with a pearlized, shimmery finish. Shine reflects light, which will make your lips look instantly plumper.

790 CLEVER CUPID

For a fuller-looking top lip, apply a highlighter or pale pink lip pencil to your Cupid's bow (the 'm' shape right above your upper lip).

791 TAKE A LIGHTER APPROACH

If you have a small mouth, avoid dark lipsticks or glosses as they can make your lips look smaller. Instead, choose a lighter shade to give the illusion of fullness.

782 CAST A SHADOW

Dot a tiny amount of soft-brown eyeliner under your lower lip line. This creates the illusion that your full lips are creating a shadow. But remember a little goes a long way – use too much and you risk looking like you're growing a beard!

fake a boob job

783 DRESS TO IMPRESS

A pretty fitted top with a narrow V-neck will accentuate a small bust. Ruffles, lace, breast pockets and wide collars will also give the illusion of larger breasts. But stay away from tops that are too big or flowing, or those with deep V-necks if you have a very small bust.

784 KEEP THEM CROSSED

Buy a multiway bra and position the straps so they cross over at the back. This will pull up your breasts and make them look larger.

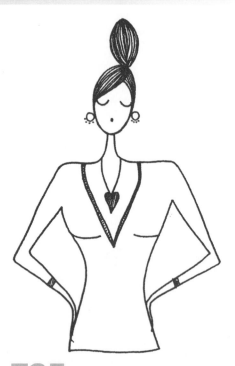

785 ENHANCE YOUR ASSETS

Padded and push-up bras obviously enhance your bust and most men will never notice the effect as all breasts look different without a bra. Don't be tempted to go for ridiculous amounts of padding, though, or you do risk disappointing your partner!

796 CLEVER CAMOUFLAGE

To make your breasts appear fuller and rounder, use a large brush to apply bronzer in back and forth strokes over the curve at the top of your breast. Then, using a thinner brush, apply a paler powder to the centre of your cleavage.

797 ENHANCING EXERCISE

To enlarge the pectoral muscles under the breast tissue, put your hands in front of your chest in a praying position. Lift your elbows up and out and push your hands together really hard for a count of 20. Repeat ten times daily.

798 MAXIMIZING MASSAGE

For plumper breasts on a night out, massage all around them with a bust cream to get the blood circulation flowing.

799 BE UPFRONT

If you're wearing a top you want to enhance your cleavage in, choose a bra that fastens at the front. This allows you to push your breasts up and closer together more easily.

fake a tummy tuck

800 PERFECT POSTURE

Straighten up and pull your stomach muscles in towards your spine – your figure will instantly look sleeker. Plus, when your posture is good you're automatically engaging and toning your stomach muscles.

801 MAGIC KNICKERS

Gripper knickers have revolutionized the underwear industry. Never before has underwear had the power to slim and smooth your belly. If you need to hide a muffin-top then go for entire body shapers.

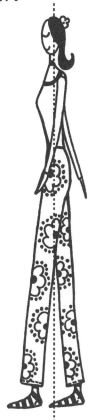

802 BE A CLING-ON

For an instantly smoother silhouette, wrap cling film (plastic wrap) around your tummy and thighs before going for a jog or working out. The sweating effect this triggers will temporarily reduce water retention and banish bloating – a fabulous quick fix if you need to squeeze into that little black dress.

803 BLOAT-BUSTING EPSOM

Epsom salts are commonly used by naturopaths and osteopaths to ease stress and flush out toxins, but they are also one of the cheapest, simplest ways to reduce tummy swelling. Buy at the pharmacy and dissolve a large handful in hot bath water.

804 SHAPING SQUATS

Squat up and down, touching the ground with your fingers, as fast as you can for a minute. This causes an oxygen deficit within your body, which forces your body to burn fat for energy. And, because it's close to the heart, fat from your middle will be the first to go.

805 JUMP FOR FLAT-STOMACH JOY

Invest in a mini-home trampoline. Bouncing on one in short five-minute bursts with ten-minute breaks in between helps tone weak tummy muscles.

806 DRINK YOURSELF THIN

Being dehydrated causes the body to store excess water, which can lead you to carry up to 1.75 kg (4 lb) of excess weight around your middle. Try to drink six to eight glasses of water daily to prevent this.

easy flu busters

807 CONCEAL REDNESS

Blowing your nose will take off any make-up so it's pointless applying foundation to this area. Instead apply concealer with a lip brush to disguise redness and reapply light touch-ups as needed. Don't bother with powder as you're probably looking pale anyway and this will make matters worse.

808 COLD CLEANSING

If your skin has dried out you'll want to slough off any flakes, but you'll need to be gentle to avoid further upsetting sore skin. You don't need a special product to do this; just gently rub your nose and lips with a facecloth soaked in warm water. Pat dry and moisturize.

809 BOOSTING BLUSH

Your complexion will look dull when you have a cold, so always wear a little more blusher than normal. But stay away from bronzers as they can look yellow on washed-out skin, making you look poorly rather than glowing.

810 GO FOR THE GLOW

Colds tend to dry out your skin so if you've got a sniffle be sure to slather on moisturizer for an instantly healthier-looking complexion and to keep nose and mouth areas from looking sore.

811 TREAD LIGHTLY

Only apply a light coat of foundation if you've got a cold. Or better still, use tinted moisturizer. Your skin will be dehydrated so too much make-up will just looked caked on.

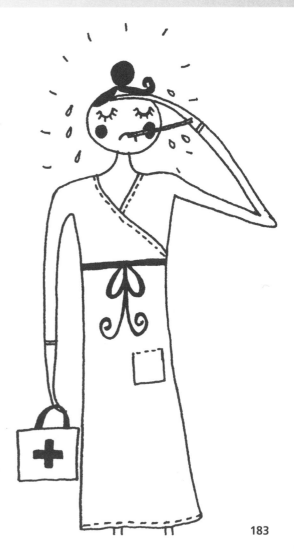

812 HERBAL HELPER

To soothe swelling under your eyes, boil 1 tablespoon of basil, 2 tablespoons of camomile, 1 tablespoon of dill and a cup of water together in a pan. Leave for five minutes (or until cool), strain and apply to the eyes using cotton pads.

813 SOOTHE A SORE NOSE

Endless nose blowing can leave your nose and lips sore and chapped. Apply petroleum jelly to your nose and lips as an overnight treatment to soothe chapped skin.

814 LUSH LIPS

Vibrant-coloured lips will really lift your face and draw attention away from a sore nose. To avoid flakiness make sure you apply lots of lip balm first, and stay away from matt shades or dull tones.

815 A SIGHT FOR SORE EYES

Apply a taupe eyeshadow from your lash line across to the crease of your eye to hide any redness. Avoid purple or blue shades as these will accentuate bloodshot eyes.

816 ACCENTUATE YOUR LASHES

If your eyelids are swollen and puffy your eyes can look tiny, but there's no need to overcompensate with loads of eye make-up. Simply curl your upper eyelashes and apply a single coat of mascara to open your eyes without upsetting sensitive skin.

disguise a sleepless night

817 WHITE OUT

A great way to hide tired eyes is to dab a shimmery white eyeshadow at the inner corners of your eyes. You'll instantly look more alert. Bright lipstick will distract attention away from your eyes.

818 LIFTING LINER

Apply white or gold eyeliner to the inner rims of your eyelids to lift your tired complexion and open up your eyes.

hide a hangover

819 IT'S A COVER-UP

Fake a restful night's sleep by using a yellow-based concealer to neutralize any redness or darkness under your eyes. Choose a concealer that's one or two shades lighter than your foundation for a brightening effect.

820 REFRESH TIRED SKIN

To re-energize your complexion and get rid of creases caused by a sleep-deprived night, apply a thick layer of facial moisturizer, then step into a hot shower. The combination of the moisturizer and the heat will plump and soften your skin.

821 WIDE-AWAKE EYES

To battle puffiness and get more out of your eye cream, store it in the refrigerator overnight. Alternatively, lie down and apply some cucumber slices straight out of the refrigerator.

822 BRUSH AWAY THE BREWERY

No one wants to smell of booze the next day but your mouth, especially your tongue, holds onto the smell of alcohol. As well as thoroughly brushing your teeth, and not forgetting your tongue, chewing a few sprigs of parsley is a great way to neutralize alcohol breath.

823 IT'S BEST TO BATHE

No matter how late you are for work, always take five minutes to have a shower. This will revitalize dull, dehydrated skin and remove the smell of alcohol from your pores.

824 SPEEDY HAIR STYLES

You probably haven't got up early enough to wash your hair before you leave the house, so don't forget to spritz on dry shampoo – an essential hair saver that's worth the money. Alternatively, put your hair up or in a ponytail, away from your face, and decorate with a hairband or scarf.

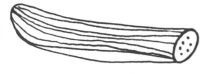

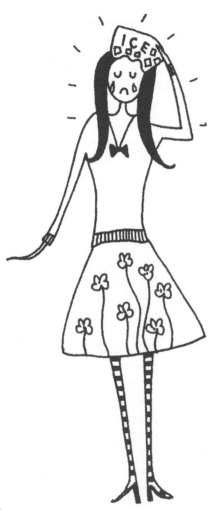

825 SHOCK YOUR SKIN

The best remedy for a puffy face is an ice bath. Ice reduces swelling, so fill a bowl with water and two trays of ice cubes and immerse your face. It will be a shock but you have to suffer for beauty!

826 COLOUR IS KEY

Your skin can look sallow and grey after a night of heavy drinking. So to avoid looking as rough as you feel, put on some brightening skin serum, pink lip colour and blusher before you leave the house.

827 WATER WORKS

Alcohol is extremely dehydrating, so the morning after you'll be suffering from a headache and dry skin. To soothe both, swap your regular coffee for a pint of boiled, warm water with the juice of half a lemon.

828 SOFTER EYES

If your eyes are bloodshot ditch your normal black mascara or eyeliner for a softer navy colour as this will emphasize the whites of your eyes.

829 HIDE THE EVIDENCE

Last night's make-up leftovers and dry skin are both telltale signs that you partied a little too hard. So use a gentle eye make-up remover to thoroughly remove mascara from under your eyes and mix a handful of oatmeal with your cleanser to gently deflake your skin.

830 TRY SPOONING

Before heading out for a big night, remember to put a couple of teaspoons in the freezer. If your eyes feel tight and tired the next morning, lie down and place one over each eye. The cooling sensation is great for soothing a pounding head, too!

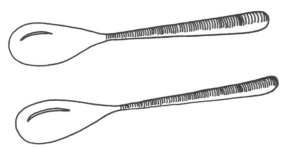

831 GLOW FOR BROKE

The morning after is not the time to recreate your sultry, heavily made-up look from last night. To look fresh faced and lift your complexion, stick to pinky tones on eyes and lips. Reds will just emphasize how washed out you are.

budget treatments for a cold sore

832 KEEP IT CLEAN

Don't use a make-up brush or concealer stick when applying cosmetics to your cold sore as you could contaminate the tools and risk spreading the infection. Use a cotton bud (swab) instead, which you can simply throw away.

833 MINT IDEA

If you feel the familiar tingle that tells you a cold sore is on its way, kick the virus without buying a treatment by applying some fresh, crushed mint leaves instead. Mint has natural antiviral properties.

834 MIRACULOUS MYRRH

Once your cold sore has appeared don't waste money on ineffective store-bought creams. Simply mix together a few drops of tea tree oil and myrrh to heal the blister.

835 EMERGENCY MEASURES

A great way to clear up a cold sore without using special creams is to dab some perfume on it. It will sting a little but the alcohol will act as an antiseptic and encourage it to dry up quickly.

836 CLEVER CONCEALING

Rub a protective coat of petroleum jelly on your cold sore before dabbing concealer on top. The petroleum jelly helps the make-up adhere to the smooth topcoat, not the dry scab underneath.

837 THE ART OF DISTRACTION

Draw people's attention away from your cold sore by applying a neutral shade of lipstick and accentuating your eyes with more dramatic make-up.

when you're pushed for time

838 FOLLOW THE RULES

Everyone knows you should emphasize either the lips or the eyes, but never both. If you're in a hurry, choose the lips, as they are easier to apply than eyes. Choose a strong-coloured lipstick to look groomed with the minimum amount of effort and money.

839 REMEMBER TO BREATHE

Tired people often have paler faces. Five minutes of deep breathing into the stomach and lungs will increase your circulation, enhancing your skin tone for a healthy glow.

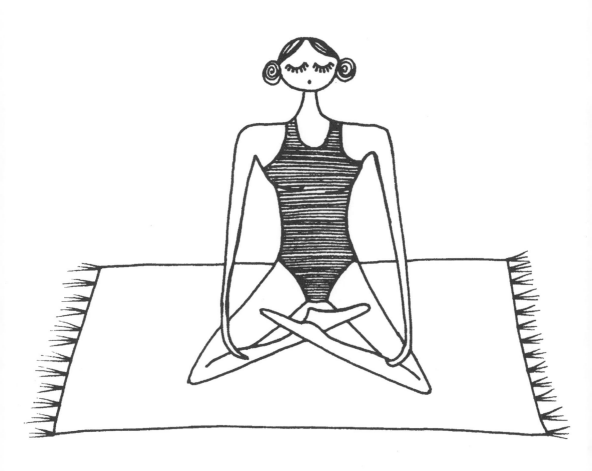

840 DRY-CLEAN HAIR

Dry shampoo sprays are a lifesaver for limp morning locks. They help to soak up grease and also add a pleasant scent. A quick spritz, a little fluff and you're good to go.

841 BRING ON THE BLUSH

When there's no time for a full-on face, just grab your blusher. Brush it on your cheeks and eyelids to lift your complexion, and you can also use it to stain your lips with a drop of water mixed in.

842 DOUBLE-DUTY BASE

Mix a little foundation into your facial moisturizer. This will allow you to moisturize and even out your skin tone at the same time – saving minutes and cash.

843 DRAW THE LINE

Don't waste time trying to get the perfect straight line of eyeliner around your eyes. Just apply a little eyeliner to the outer corners of your eyes to accentuate them in less than half the time.

844 ORDER IT

Simply knowing the fastest way to apply your standard make-up can cut down on the time you spend – and save money on expensive SOS products. First apply foundation, then a powder blusher (it's easier to apply than cream), then simple eye make-up. Finally, apply a coat gloss to your lips.

845 LET'S NOT BE HASTY

Stay calm – panic will cause you to make make-up mistakes, which means you'll spend longer doing it and will require the use of more products to fix.

846 DON'T DOUBLE UP

One coat of mascara is sufficient. You can also save time and make the tube last longer by only applying it to the top lashes.

847 FAST FINGERS

Rub foundation between your hands then apply with just your fingertips. The heat helps it spread faster, which means you'll need less and apply it more evenly.

home detox

848 SUPER SMOOTHIE

You can make a week's worth of detox smoothie for the price of one glass from a juice bar. Choose a high-fibre fruit, such as apple or pear, add a citrus fruit to cleanse your digestive tract, then oatmeal or wheatgerm to help eliminate toxins.

849 FEELING FLUSH?

The basic principle of any detox is to drink enough each day to help your body flush out toxins. You need to drink at least 2 litres (4½ US pints) of liquid a day. Choose water, herbal tea or very diluted vegetable juice.

850 BUY A BLENDER

Invest in a juicer or hand blender to make spa-standard detox juices and smoothies. You can get a blender relatively cheaply, so don't feel you need to go for a top-of-the-range one. But do opt for one that's easy to clean, or your passion for juicing will quickly fade.

851 DETOX DRINK

If you've been overindulging in alcohol, you need to eliminate harmful toxins, which can dull and dry your skin. Start your day with a glass of boiled, warm water containing a slice of lemon to jump-start your liver and help balance your body's pH level.

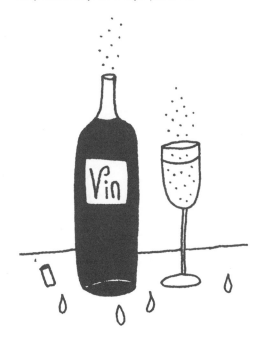

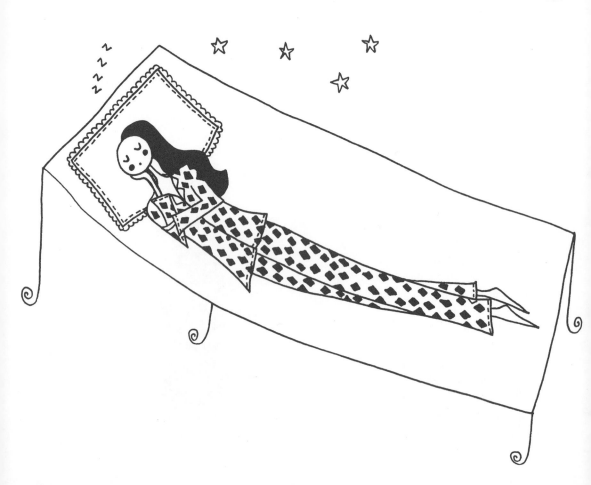

852 SOOTHING SHUT-EYE

At any spa the importance of sleep is to be stressed. Make sure you get the eight hours you need by sprinkling a few drops of lavender oil onto your pillow.

853 DON'T BE GREEN

Why pay top dollar for a green tea-infused detox product when you can get the real thing for a fraction of the price? Simply guzzle down three to five cups a day for the same natural antioxidant effects.

854 BE YOUR OWN DIET DOC

For a home-detox diet, load up on fruit, veggies and wholegrains, such as super-cleansing brown rice. Avoid red meat, caffeine, alcohol, sugar, salt, processed foods and anything containing artificial additives.

855 VITAL VEG

You can create your own blend of detoxifying vegetable juice for a fraction of what they charge you at health-food stores. Try juicing a mix of beetroot, ginger, celery, parsley and carrots.

856 GIVE YOUR LIVER A LIFT

Make your own liver-cleansing treatment, rather than buying fancy detox formulas. Squeeze the juice of a grapefruit and a lemon into a glass of water. Using a garlic press, squeeze in two cloves of garlic and a knob of fresh ginger. Add 1 tablespoon of olive oil. Mix thoroughly and sip slowly.

857 BREATHE EASY

Do you really need to pay someone to teach you how to breathe? To help you eliminate toxins try this cleansing yoga breath. Inhale slowly and deeply, then, exhale briskly, as if you were sneezing. Continue for as long as you feel comfortable, but stop if you feel light-headed.

858 WORK IT OUT

Exercise is an important part of a detox, as it increases your blood circulation and lymphatic flow. This helps reduce fluid retention and encourages the lymphatic system to eliminate toxins. A brisk walk each morning of your detox will work as well as an exercise class.

859 SWAP JAVA FOR JUICE

Instead of your normal store-bought latte, reach for a homemade fruit juice in the morning. Consumed on an empty stomach, fruit acids are very effective detoxifiers. Pineapple is a great choice, as it contains natural enzymes that aid digestion.

860 JUST ADD SALT

Dead sea salts are a detox retreat favourite but you can buy a bag for next to nothing at your local health-food store. Add a big handful to your bath water. Hot water draws toxins to the skin's surface and, as the water cools, it pulls the toxins away from the skin. The salt enhances this detoxification process.

861 DETOX-FRIENDLY DIET

There's no need to pay out for a book on detox diets. Putting together a menu for yourself is easy. Start the day with a smoothie or porridge, have a fish salad or stuffed peppers for lunch and in the evening enjoy soup or a vegetable stir-fry with brown rice.

862 MINIMAL MAKE-UP

At a retreat or spa you'd be encouraged to go cosmetic-free but you can also do this in your own home. Go without make-up for a whole weekend – let your skin breathe and have a break from chemicals.

863 MIX IT UP

If the healthy meals you're cooking seem bland don't splash out for pre-prepared detox food, just add spice with aromatic herbs. Basil is good for digestion, parsley is rich in vitamin C and rosemary stimulates the whole body, or check out Ayurvedic recipes at www.joyfulbelly.com.

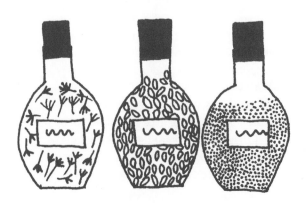

864 TOXIC TONGUE

A great home-detox treatment is to use the back of a spoon or a dry toothbrush to scrape your tongue. Toxins from the body accumulate on the top of your tongue and scraping is an effective way of preventing them re-entering your system.

865 SWEAT-TEA

Sweating helps rid your body of toxins, but rather than splash out on a sauna or Turkish bath, just run yourself a hot bath and drink a herbal tea such as elderberry, sarsaparilla or lungwort to encourage you to sweat.

866 LET NATURE LIFT YOUR SPIRIT

A common feature of retreats is that they are in the countryside, but you don't need to pay to enjoy the benefits of fresh air. Simply head to a local park or beauty spot.

867 SKIN PURIFICATION

Detox retreats include treatments to help remove impurities from your skin. Add two cups of apple cider vinegar to warm bath water for a deeply detoxifying soak.

sun-protection savings

868 SENSITIVE SUNBLOCK

Don't pay extra for a specialized sunscreen if you have sensitive skin. Just shop around for one with a very simple ingredients list, containing only the physical ingredients zinc oxide or titanium dioxide. Unlike chemical sunscreen agents, which absorb UV rays, it's rare to have an allergy to physical sunscreens.

869 AVOID BREAKOUTS

You don't need an expensive oil-free sunscreen to prevent breakouts; just look for one that is water or gel based. It's a bonus if you can find one that is fragrance-free.

870 SENSIBLE SPFS

You should always wear at least SPF 15 to protect your skin. So anything with an SPF lower than this is a waste of money when it comes to preventing skin damage or premature ageing.

871 TWO FOR ONE

Make sure you buy a 'broad spectrum' sunscreen that protects you from both UVA and UVB rays. You really need to protect against both so there's no point buying a bottle that only shields your skin from one.

872 DON'T OVERSTOCK

Sunscreen doesn't last very long – heat and bacteria damage it over time. Don't be tempted to bulk-buy when you see special offers unless you know you're going to use it. Discard any that is past the expiration date.

873 INSPECT THE INGREDIENTS

Sunscreen doesn't need to be expensive to be effective. As long as zinc oxide, titanium dioxide or avobenzone are listed as ingredients you should be in safe hands.

874 MULTIPURPOSE MOISTURIZER

If you prefer the shade and don't plan to expose a lot of skin to the sun you can swap sunscreen for an inexpensive facial moisturizer with an SPF. Apply to your face, neck and hands every day.

875 BUY BEFORE YOU FLY

Stores in popular tourist destinations tend to bump up the price of sunscreen as they know they will have a captive audience. Buy before you fly to save a little cash.

876 EARLY APPLICATION

Why spend money on a product that isn't going to work because you don't use it properly? Follow the golden sunscreen rule, which means applying half an hour before you go out in the sun for it to be effective.

877 BE GENEROUS

Don't be stingy when applying sunscreen. For this reason, it's better to buy a cheap (but effective) sunscreen, as you won't need to worry about how much you slather on.

878 HERE'S THE RUB...

Even waterproof sunscreen can't withstand towel-drying so always reapply sunscreen after drying yourself, or alternatively let yourself air-dry. Either way, treatment for sunburn will cost far more than using enough sunscreen.

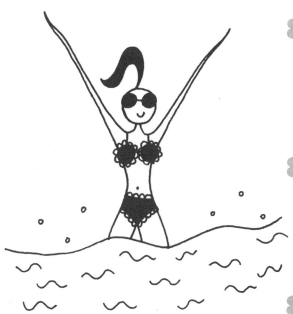

880 LIFESAVER

If sunscreen starts to smell funny or separates, you should get rid of it because it won't work properly. However, you can prolong the life of your sunscreen by storing it in the refrigerator and keeping it in the shade while you're on the beach.

881 AFTER SUN

It's important to moisturize your skin after sun exposure, but don't feel the need to buy expensive after-sun products – normal moisturizers or body lotions will work just as well. Add a dollop of aloe vera gel to soothe sore skin.

882 PRICELESS PRODUCT

The only skincare product that can slow the ageing process, reduce scarring and acne, all but eliminate wrinkles and even prevent cancer, is sunscreen. When you consider the amount of money spent on plastic surgery and cosmetics, it's a wonder why anyone wouldn't use sunscreen daily. It's the most important and cost-effective part of your skincare routine.

879 IN THE SWIM

If you are going swimming make sure your sunscreen won't wash off the second you hit the water. Generally, a sunscreen that is 'water repellent' will withstand two 20-minute swims. While one that is 'waterproof' will withstand four 20-minute dips. Check the details on the bottle you buy.

cut-price celebrity secrets

883 STRAWBERRY SMILE

Catherine Zeta-Jones supposedly owes her perfect smile to homemade strawberry toothpaste. Strawberries contain natural fruit acids, which act as a mild astringent when mashed up and mixed with bicarbonate of soda (baking soda).

884 SUPERMODEL SKIN

The original supermodel, Cindy Crawford, keeps her skin super-moist by mixing some milk in with the water she spritzes on her face during the day.

885 OIL COMES IN HANDY

Save yourself the cost of a professional manicure by stealing Julia Roberts' nail secret. The actress soaks her nails in olive oil, which moisturizes without weakening them. The oil also softens cuticles and prevents hangnails.

886 THE OLD TOOTHPASTE TRICK

Dab some toothpaste onto spots (pimples) and leave overnight. Jennifer Love Hewitt is a fan of this trick.

887 HEALTHY HAIR

If you're planning a baby, or just had one, you could take a leaf out of Gwyneth Paltrow's haircare book. The actress swears that nothing has ever kept her long blonde locks in better condition than prenatal vitamins, so she carried on taking them post-birth.

888 BAIN DU VIN

Got some red wine left over from the night before? You could use it to copy *Desperate Housewives'* star Teri Hatcher, who apparently pours two glasses into her bath water! Red wine contains resveratrol, which can firm the skin and improve elasticity.

889 BEAUTIFUL BABY, BEAUTIFUL BODY

She may be 'Posh' but for her 'everyday body moisturizer' Mrs Beckham swears by nothing more fancy than baby oil.

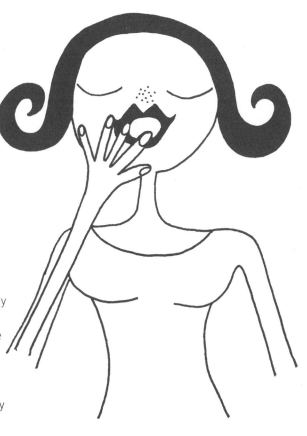

890 SEXY POUT SECRET

Mariah Carey's fulsome pout is not the result of any expensive treatment or even pricey lipstick. The singer simply applies a touch of peppermint extract to her lips, which naturally increases the blood flow.

891 BUTTER YOURSELF BETTER

Cocoa butter is both cheap and versatile according to Minnie Driver, who uses the vitamin E-enriched cream on her skin and to tame her curly locks.

892 MAGIC POWDER

The secret to Angelina Jolie's amazing hair is apparently a sprinkling of baby powder. Her hairstylist adds volume by rubbing powder into her roots and then blow-drying it away. The powder also mops up excess grease.

893 WORKS INSIDE AND OUT

Singer and actress Hilary Duff apparently keeps a spray bottle of mint tea in the refrigerator. Cold mint tea both cools the skin and stimulates blood flow.

894 COFFEE TO GO

Forget expensive cellulite creams. Oscar-winning actress Halle Berry allegedly mixes coffee grounds into her body wash to keep her rear looking smooth and firm.

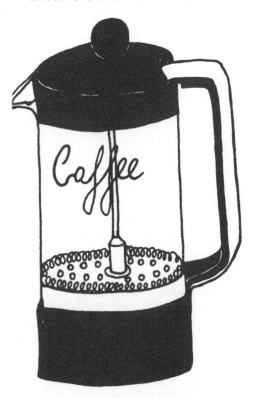

895 BEAUTY OF THE BALM

J-Lo is said to be a big fan of the versatility of plain old lip balm – she uses it to add shine, smooth hair and to remove make-up.

896 ACHIEVE NATURAL WAVES

Ever wondered how Jessica Alba gets those great natural waves in her hair? She applies a leave-in conditioner and wraps her hair in a bun until it dries. Then, she simply lets it out. The waves get less puffy over time, so your hair looks even better the next day.

897 FORGET FANCY STUFF

Stunning singer Gwen Stefani is in no doubt about what works best as a moisturizer – she has said she prefers baby lotion to any fancy products.

898 EYE CONTACT

Run out of your favourite eyeshadow? Well, the secret behind Charlize Theron's stunning eyes is apparently bronze shimmer lip gloss. Her make-up artist adds a dab right above the eyelashes and then uses a finger to blend.

899 PROUD TO BE PALE

To keep her famously pale skin looking young and fresh Australian actress Nicole Kidman relies on one trick above all others – she stays out of the sun. It's simple, it's free and it works!

900 WATER, WATER EVERYWHERE

The key active ingredient in Naomi Campbell's beauty regime is H_2O. The supermodel says she drinks 'loads and loads' of water every day, especially if she has to fly somewhere.

901 LIKE MOTHER LIKE DAUGHTER

American Beauty actress Mena Suvari keeps her skin rose-petal soft by applying aloe vera gel after cleansing her face – a regime she copied from her mother.

902 WONDERS OF NATURE

Bollywood superstar and former Miss World Aishwarya Rai drinks hot water with lemon and honey every morning to keep her skin clear. She also favours cucumber as a natural eye compress.

903 LIPS AS SWEET AS CANDY

Former *Friends* actress Jennifer Aniston has a sweet trick for super-soft lips. She combines a small amount of sugar and water in a teaspoon and applies it to her lips with a toothbrush. Gently scrub in for truly kissable lips.

904 WHY BOTHER WITH BLUSHER?

Cameron Diaz doesn't bother buying blusher. Instead, the former model uses a trick from her high-fashion photography days and uses her lipstick as blush, giving her cheeks a youthful, dewy glow. It also ensures that her cheeks match her lips.

905 HINT TO TINT

Porcelain Australian beauty Cate Blanchett prefers to have her eyelashes tinted rather than have one more daily make-up chore to worry about. Follow her lead and you will not only save on mascara, but dreaded 'panda eyes' will become a thing of the past.

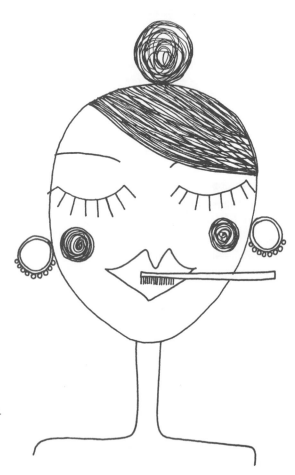

906 COOL HAIRDO

Liv Tyler's hairstylist uses a fresh-from-the-freezer ice cube and rubs it up and down the hair shaft to create shine. The ice cube chills the hair, thus sealing the cuticle, which makes hair gleam.

907 DON'T OVERDO IT

Uma Thurman swears by a simple make-up commandment that also happens to be a good cost-saving tip: less is more. The stunning actress usually wears just concealer, mascara and lip gloss.

908 DO IT YOURSELF

If you think that a special occasion automatically means paying for a salon visit, then you may be interested to know that Beyoncé's make-up artist of choice for many red carpet events is herself!

909 SECRET TO LASTING BEAUTY

Like any true Italian, Sophia Loren loves olive oil. Not only does the screen legend make sure she gets enough in her diet, she rubs a small amount in her skin everyday.

910 CHERRY ON TOP

German supermodel Claudia Schiffer has been known to wear an unusual but delicious lip tint – cherry gelatine! Dip a damp cotton bud (swab) into the flavoured powder and drag it across your moist lips. Leave it on for five minutes, then lick it off. Top with some gloss and you're done.

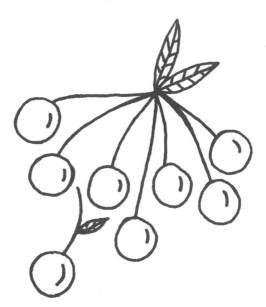

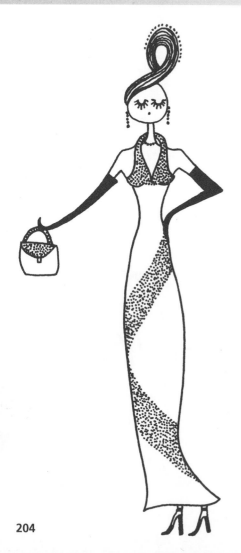

911 STYLIST, WHAT STYLIST?

The Oscar-winning actress Helen Mirren is said to save money on stylists by cutting her own hair. Apparently she gets her hubbie to snip the back bits she can't reach!

912 THE EYES HAVE IT

Tyra Banks, the former supermodel turned presenter, believes that the very best eye cream you can use is none other than petroleum jelly. She has even called the household basic her 'number one beauty secret'.

913 ALWAYS BE PREPARED

Sexy and sensible actress Scarlett Johansson always has cotton buds (swabs) in her handbag for correcting unexpected make-up disasters. Keep some with you whenever you're out and you won't have to worry about constant reapplication or, worse, washing off and starting again.

914 REMEMBER TO REMOVE

Christina Aguilera performed all through her teens so she certainly knows the value of keeping your skin clear. Her number one tip? Never go to sleep without washing your face – after all, prevention is cheaper than paying for a cure.

915 SLEEP RIGHT

Now in her late forties, TV star Heather Locklear keeps her skin wrinkle-free by looking after it in her sleep. She never sleeps on her stomach and always makes sure the sheets are silky and soft.

understand advertising

916 WORKS AT A CELLULAR LEVEL

Any product that exfoliates dead cells from the surface layer of your skin, exposing the underlying skin cells, could claim it works on a 'cellular level'. Therefore, any cheap exfoliator will do the same job.

917 FOR 'SUPERFICIAL LINES'

'Superficial lines' refers to the temporary lines caused by dryness, not wrinkles. Superficial lines will disappear when you put on any moisturizer.

918 OIL-FREE PRODUCTS

Being oil-free doesn't guarantee that a product won't clog pores and cause spots (pimples). Similarly, not all oils are bad for oily or acne-prone skin. Certain oils, like tea tree, help clear acne and balance the skin's natural oils. Look for non-comedogenic instead, which means it's been shown not to block pores in tests.

919 FOR THE DELICATE EYE AREA

There's no reason an eye cream can't be used on the face or that face lotion can't be used around the eyes. The ingredients of these products are rarely different enough to warrant the extra expense of buying a separate moisturizer for each area. Extra-rich night creams could irritate eyes though.

920 BOTANICAL PRODUCTS

This doesn't mean the product is chemical-free or natural. Most botanical products are a mixture of both plant and chemical ingredients. And just because something is botanical doesn't mean it's automatically good for your skin.

921 PATENTED PRODUCTS

This just means that the company was able to show that a formula or ingredient was in some way unique. It doesn't mean it works. A company could patent a terrible formula as well as a good formula.

922 DERMATOLOGIST TESTED

This doesn't actually tell you a whole lot about the product – only that it's had the basic necessary testing. It certainly doesn't mean that it'll be any better for your skin than a cheaper product. Feel free to ignore.

923 CONTAINS NATURAL INGREDIENTS

This just means that the ingredients were not produced chemically in a lab. Instead they were extracted from plants or animals. However, it doesn't mean that it won't cause allergic reactions. In fact, some natural ingredients are very common causes of allergies.

924 REJUVENATING CREAMS

A rejuvenating product won't necessarily make you look younger. Basically, any product can claim to rejuvenate your skin because it's a subjective term and there's no way to prove whether it does or not.

925 DESIGNED ESPECIALLY FOR YOUR SKIN

Well that's great, but what exactly is it designed to do? Vague phrases like this don't actually tell you anything about what the product will do for you.

926 LEAVES SKIN FEELING SMOOTHER

Beware of the word 'feeling' in beauty advertising. 'Feeling' is a subjective word, so it's very hard to prove whether or not the product does what it claims to do.

927 PENETRATES THE DERMAL LAYER

'Epidermal' refers to the top layers of the skin and 'dermal' means the skin's deepest layer. All these words really mean is that the product is absorbed by your skin – which should be true of all skincare products.

928 REPAIRING

Another vague term that means nothing – just because a product promises to 'repair' your skin doesn't mean it will be any more effective than a cheaper moisturizer.

929 DETOXIFYING

This is really just another word for cleansing. Good old soap and water could be said to have a 'detoxifying' effect on your skin!

930 LABORATORY TESTED

But where was it tested? If the research was conducted by the company's own lab, it can't be considered as unbiased.

big claims, little benefits

931 CLOSES YOUR PORES

It's impossible to actually close skin pores. Pores are skin openings that allow sebum to flow to the surface to keep skin supple. If your pores are enlarged you can lessen their appearance simply by exfoliating.

932 REMOVES BLACKHEADS

Any lotion that claims to remove blackheads won't work. The only way to remove blackheads is by squeezing, but even then the pore will usually fill with oil again overnight and the pesky blackhead will return within a day or two.

933 TREATS WRINKLES FROM THE INSIDE

Creams don't reach the lower skin layers in the same way cosmetic filler injections do. So while they may plump up wrinkles on the surface of the skin, they cannot work within the skin to smooth them.

934 RESURFACES THE SKIN

No skincare product can completely resurface your skin. All exfoliating products will remove a top layer of dead cells from the surface of your skin, but none have the power to actually create a new surface. Besides, that would really hurt!

935 DEEPER CLEANSE

No cleanser can get more deeply inside your pores than another – so don't pay more for it. Cleansers can only clean the surface of your skin.

936 REDUCES CELLULITE

Any product you apply to the surface of your skin can't reduce the fatty tissue that causes the dimples on your thighs. They may temporarily smooth its appearance, but they cannot 'treat' the actual cellulite.

937 REVITALIZES 'LIFELESS' HAIR

Hair is 'lifeless' because it is life-less. Your hair is dead and no amount of product is going to change this. Thin hair, however, can have volume added.

938 HAS A LIFTING EFFECT ON YOUR SKIN

No cream can fight gravity! It can add moisture and may also increase firmness, but lift skin it cannot do.

939 SPEEDS CELL GROWTH

Even if scientists had managed to find an effective way to speed skin cell growth, you're unlikely to be able to buy something that powerful in a jar at the beauty counter.

940 BOOSTS NAIL GROWTH

Your nails are dead so applying a product to them in the form of a varnish or lotion is unlikely to be able to speed up their growth. However, products can protect nails and keep them from breaking, which may mean they get longer quicker.

941 MOISTURIZES FOR 24 HOURS

This lab-based claim may sound impressive but it's unlikely that any cream making this boast has been rigorously tested on real people – with all skin types, living a normal day that includes showers, gym workouts and make-up removal.

942 LENGTHENS LASHES

No mascara can actually add length – it can only thicken and make lashes look longer by coating with colour from the root to the often lighter tip. Don't pay extra for this promise.

943 CONTOURS YOUR BODY

This implies that the product changes the appearance of the skin or the body's shape – but under FDA rules 'restructuring' skin, or having an effect on fat deposits, means that it's a drug and has to go through extensive and expensive clinical trials. Treat this claim with caution.

944 WON'T IRRITATE YOUR SKIN

Even if a product has undergone intensive testing, it's always possible that even a gentle product can irritate some users, due to allergies or misuse.

945 MAKE YOUR HAIR TWO-TIMES STRONGER

Beware big claims such as these, for how can you possibly measure how much stronger a product has made your hair?

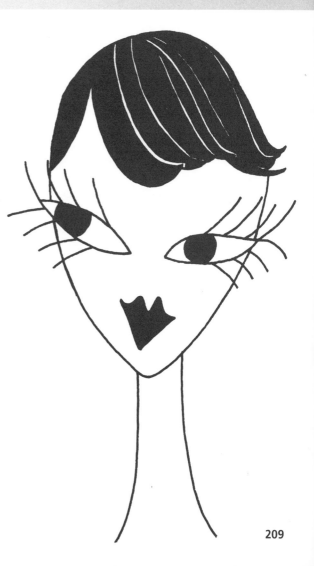

be savvy about skin supplements

946 A TASTE OF THE SEA

Over 100 minerals are available in sea salt. Throw away any refined table salt in your home and replace it with natural sea salt and you will get a large proportion of the minerals your body needs without buying any tablets. (Avoid too much salt if you have high blood pressure.)

947 DON'T FLUSH IT AWAY

If they're not taken properly, supplements can be flushed through your body without being absorbed. So don't waste your tablets. Take them with room-temperature water – hot or chilled drinks can damage them. Always read the label on the bottle and take supplements as directed.

948 CHEAP WORKS JUST AS WELL

All vitamins are essentially the same, so buy the cheapest ones you can find.

949 MAKE FOOD FIRST CHOICE

Supplements can't replace food nor undo the damage caused by bad eating habits. So make sure you're eating a healthy, balanced diet before you splash the cash on any supplements.

950 CHECK THE EXPIRY DATE

Vitamin tablets don't last forever. When buying them, steer clear of supplements within six to nine months of their expiration dates. They've probably been in the bottle for several years and may be past their prime.

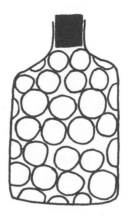
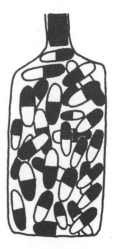

when to spend: the hits

951 COD LIVER OIL

Any omega-3-loaded fish oil will help maintain and build supple skin, lustrous hair and stronger nails. It can also help improve the texture of bumpy skin on the tops of your arms.

952 PROTEIN POWER

Studies have shown biotin supplements can strengthen dry, brittle nails, making them a worthwhile beauty investment.

953 LOTTA BOTTLE

Research by Swedish scientists has found that yogurt and yogurt-type digestion-improving drinks – the type that contain friendly bacteria known as probiotics – do work and also boost the immune system. A bottle a day should leave you less bloated and looking and feeling more energized.

954 MAGNESIUM OK

Women are often low in this mineral, so a supplement can help ease PMS symptoms and reduce monthly skin breakouts.

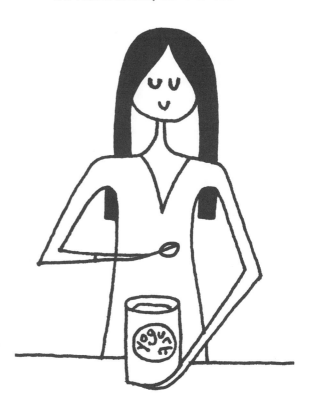

955 SUPER SILICA

This natural mineral is necessary for healthy hair, skin and nails. Taking a supplement will improve hair thickness, skin tone and nail strength. It is also widely promoted for the prevention of osteoporosis.

956 EVENING, PRIMROSE

One of the most concentrated sources of gama linoleic acid (GLA) – an essential fatty acid – is evening primrose oil. GLAs have anti-inflammatory properties and play an important role in maintaining hormone balance and healthy skin – they can help treat dry or acne-prone skin and even eczema. Evening primrose is also said to improve the condition of nails, scalp and hair, so it may be worth trying.

957 ZINC FOR ZITS

Acne is often linked to zinc deficiency. A dose of 30 mg per day can improve your skin. But get the right type – zinc picolinate is the easiest to absorb, so you may be wasting your money if you buy other forms that often pass straight through the body.

when to save: the misses

958 EAT IT UP

You only need a tiny amount of the mineral selenium and this can easily be obtained from meat, nuts, bread, fish or eggs. Taking a supplement will increase the chances of absorbing too much, which can actually lead to weaker skin, hair and nails.

959 C CLEARLY

There are no scientific studies that show that taking vitamin C as a supplement has any effect on improving skin.

960 COLLAGEN CAPSULES

As the body gets older it stops producing collagen but taking supplements won't help you regain a youthful appearance. According to the British Skin Foundation, there's no evidence to support the idea that oral collagen supplements prevent wrinkles or improve the condition of your skin.

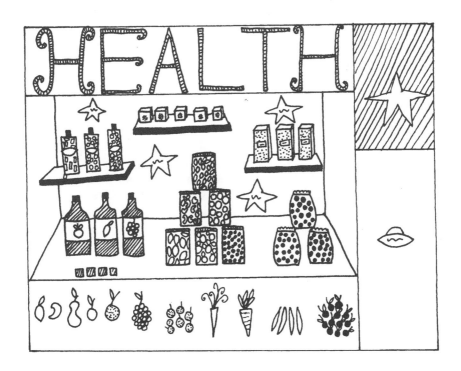

961 AIN'T NO SUNSHINE

Tan-optimizing pills aren't a great idea as they can provide a false
sense of security, meaning you end up spending longer in the
sun and causing damage to your skin. A tan is a sign of damaged
skin and there's no such thing as a safe tan. You're better off
spending your pennies on a fake tan with a high SPF built in.

962 KEEP IT REAL

There's no proof that taking synthesized supplements of single antioxidants will keep skin young. It's thought that antioxidants probably only work as part of a food as they may need other components of the food to be effective.

963 NOT A-LIST

Vitamin A (retinol) helps keep skin healthy. But a woman needs just 0.6 mg a day, according to the UK's Food Standards Agency, which means you can get all you need from foods such as cheese, eggs, oily fish, milk and yogurt. More than 1.5 mg per day may actually make your bones more brittle and prone to fracture as you age.

964 E-ASY DOES IT

Vitamin E helps protect cell membranes by acting as an antioxidant. While it may be moisturizing, taking a supplement can't actually fight ageing or prevent wrinkles.

965 B COMPLEX

While B vitamins are vital for healthy skin, hair and nails, you're better off getting your daily dose from food, as overdosing is easy and can lead to nasty side effects such as chest pain, fatigue, stomach upset, depression or numbness.

966 WATER WORKS

So-called 'beauty waters' can be a waste of money because often the vitamins or herbs they contain are in such tiny amounts they're unlikely to have any effect. Also they often contain sugar or artificial sweeteners, in which case you'd be better off having a glass of ordinary water from the tap (faucet).

967 WRINKLE RIP-OFF?

Thinking of buying an expensive anti-ageing vitamin formula? Bear in mind there's no proven research that taking a pill each day will improve wrinkles or stop them from forming.

the maybes

968 A BUNCH OF HELP

Grape-seed extract appears to preserve and reinforce collagen in the skin. However, only 28 per cent of grape-seed extract's active component remains in the body after 24 hours, so supplements must be taken at the same time daily for it to be effective.

969 TIME TO GET CO-ZY?

Coenzyme Q10 is vital for protecting skin from ageing free-radical damage, but by the time we're 40 our bodies are only producing a quarter of the amount they did in our 20s. More research needs to be done, but some experts believe they're a supplement worth spending money on.

how to haggle

970 BE COURAGEOUS

Don't be afraid to haggle, even in a department store or beauty salon chain. The worst that can happen is they say 'no'. And if you're successful you'll leave glowing with the knowledge that you just paid less than everyone else for your haircut/massage/lipstick.

971 A RIGHT CHARMER

But do remember that aggressive or forceful haggling is a mistake as it annoys the person you're dealing with. You'll get further if you're polite, charming and treat the situation with humour.

972 AVOID AN AUDIENCE

Anyone in a position to decide the price of something is usually aware that if other people are around there's a risk that they too will want a discount. So be discreet and haggle quietly to allow the person in charge to be more flexible.

215

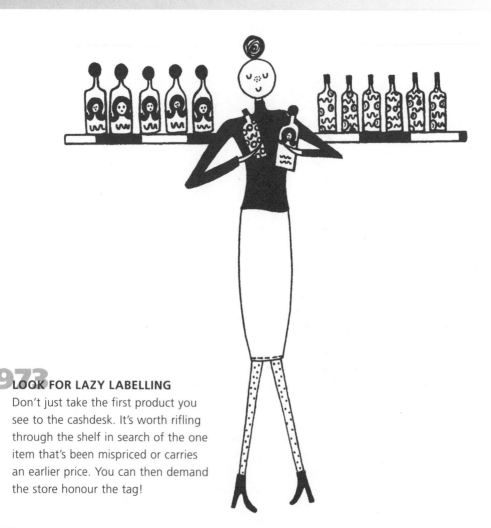

973 LOOK FOR LAZY LABELLING

Don't just take the first product you
see to the cashdesk. It's worth rifling
through the shelf in search of the one
item that's been mispriced or carries
an earlier price. You can then demand
the store honour the tag!

974 CREATE A PRICE WAR

Shop around before you haggle. If you know you can get an item or service cheaper elsewhere then tell the sales assistant/beauty therapist and they may well offer you a deal to secure your custom. The more stores you play against each other, the better your chance of bagging a bargain.

975 INTERNET INVESTIGATION

Many retailers operate online and have stores on the web, with the online price invariably being cheaper than in their individual outlets. If you print out their online price and ask them to match it in-store you can save on the delivery fee.

976 BUILD A RELATIONSHIP

If you always buy your beauty products from the same salesperson or your treatments from the same beauty therapist, you'll soon build up a friendly relationship with them. And from time to time they may reward your loyalty with freebies or a ten per cent discount.

977 DEAL WITH DECISION MAKERS

If a salesperson doesn't have the power to give you a discount, then find out who does. In chain stores, that's typically a manager or supervisor. The same holds true when you're negotiating fees for beauty treatments.

978 SHOW AN INTEREST

When buying a beauty product or receiving a beauty treatment, ask about the other products and services they offer. Ask lots of questions and show a real interest and you may be offered a free sample or trial.

979 IT'S A GIFT!

When purchasing a beauty product or perfume tell the salesperson that it's a gift. They may throw some free samples into your bag as an extra treat or at the very least offer you prettier packaging!

980 SPOT IMPERFECTIONS

Always point out any flaws in the product, for example if the packaging is damaged, and ask for a discount.

981 TIMING IS EVERYTHING

Don't try to haggle on a busy Saturday afternoon. There's no reason for a sales assistant to offer a reduction when they have plenty of other customers willing to pay full price. Weekdays and early mornings are the best time to ask for money off.

982 SUPERSIZE SALE BARGAINS

If the price is already reduced, such as during a sale, there is often greater flexibility. Sales are designed to clear room for new stock, so managers are often willing to accept lower than the marked sale price. A bit of cheeky haggling might see you being offered extra discounts.

983 SLEUTH FOR PRE-SALES

Stores rarely put all their stock on sale at once, but if some products are discounted it is always worth asking if the one you want is due to be in the sale too. Chances are the retailer may be able to sell it at sale price if you ask nicely.

984 BLAME YOUR OTHER HALF

When deciding whether to buy an extra product or treatment a good line to try is 'I would love to buy this, but my husband/boyfriend will go mad if I pay this amount'. A sales assistant who empathizes could well knock a little money off.

985 SERVICE SWAP

If you're willing to design and hand out flyers for your hairstylist or beauty therapist, they may offer you a free cut or at least a discounted rate in return for your marketing services.

986 STAY IN TOUCH

Always ask to go on the mailing list at stores and salons. This will keep you informed of any special-offer evenings or discreet deals for valued customers.

987 DON'T BE AFRAID OF SILENCE

When haggling it pays to pause. Let the sales assistant fill the gaps in the conversation with better offers.

988 BULK-BUY BARGAINING

Discounts are more often available if you're buying a lot of items in one go. So if you're going to buy a few products from the same range, or are planning to stock up on your favourite, it's always worth asking if you've earned a discount. Why not get together a few friends who are after the same thing?

989 PICK YOUR BATTLES

You're much more likely to be able to haggle for bargains in independent stores or salons than you are in major chains. Any store or salon where you can speak directly to the owner is a better bet, as they will have the authority to negotiate.

990 ASK FOR A CASH DISCOUNT

Offer to pay in cash. You may just save yourself another ten per cent. Many credit card companies charge stores a fee for every transaction they carry out, therefore some stores offer a discount on goods for a cash sale. This applies particularly to the smaller independent stores.

991 THREATEN TO QUIT

If you have a membership at a gym, or a longstanding relationship with a beauty salon, tell them that you dearly want to stay but you've seen too many better deals elsewhere, then see what they offer.

final freebies

992 SAVVY SAMPLES

When buying make-up or beauty products always insist on having a sample first. Your skin, hair and colouring are unique so you have the right to ensure that products work for you before you invest in them.

993 FRIENDLY FREEBIES

It always pays to have friends in the beauty industry. They'll often be sent more free samples than they can use, so if they're feeling generous they may let you take some off their hands.

994 VALUABLE VOUCHERS

There are many websites that offer voucher codes that you can use in stores or online. Just enter the name of the brand you are looking for and 'money off' into a search engine and you could find vouchers for free delivery or up to 20 per cent off.

995 CARRY AN EMPTY

Want to try a beauty product but they don't have a ready-to-go sample? Whip out your own container and they'll have no excuse for saying no!

996 BE PAID TO SHOP

Get a store card for the introductory offer, then pay the bill asap and cut up the card. Alternatively, use cash-back credit cards and pay off the monthly balance in full.

997 PERFECT PROMOTIONS

If you can, wait until your favourite brand is running a promotion in department stores or pharmacies. You'll often get a free bag of goodies with your purchase.

998 WATCH OUT FOR ADS

The newer the product, the greater the marketing budget, which means you're more likely to get your hands on a free sample.

999 READ ALL ABOUT IT

Keep an eye out in newspapers and magazines for reader's trial panels. You'll be sent free samples of beauty products for you to try and review.

1000 MASTER MARKET RESEARCH

Sign up to online market research companies or take part in street surveys. The researchers will often offer free samples to people who are willing to give them feedback on new products.

1001 POCKET SAMPLES

Whether you are in the hair salon or dentist's waiting room, don't pass up the opportunity to flick through glossy magazines. They often have mini hair and skin samples you can pocket. After all, why let them go to waste?

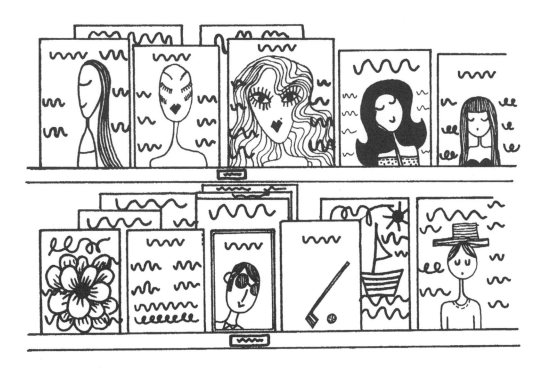

acne 212
acupuncture 152
advertising 205–9
age spots 13, 29, 80, 118
air diffuser 111
alcohol 144, 185, 186, 191, 193
allergies 206, 209
aloe vera 52, 123, 197, 201
alpha-hydroxy acids (AHAs) 37, 73, 76, 87
alpha-lipoic acid 36
anti-ageing: body massage 140; eats
    12–15; facial products 80–82; pills 214
antioxidants 12, 13, 14, 17, 19, 38, 80,
    82, 85, 87, 130, 140, 214
aromatherapy 153, 154
Ayurvedic recipes 194
Ayurvedic treatments 153, 154

baby lotion 201
baby oil 50, 199
baby powder 200
bad breath (halitosis) 129, 132
bath bombs 167
bathing: after a night drinking 185; berry
    bath 166; chocolate bliss 164, 167;
    herbal 164; vanilla bath bubbles 167
beauty colleges 161
beauty gadgets 31–5
'beauty waters' 214
beta-carotene 12
beta-hydroxy acid (BHA or salicylic acid) 37
bicarbonate of soda (baking powder) 51,
    97, 128, 164, 167
bikini trimmer 35
bioflavonoids 17
biotin 21, 211
blackheads 207
blood circulation 13, 17, 92, 138, 139,
    144, 154, 167, 181, 188, 200
blushers 28, 50, 58, 60–61, 176, 183, 190
body lotion 138, 141, 142, 197
body oil 142
body treatments, do-it-yourself 138–42
body-toning pads 31
boob job, faked 180–81

brands 23
bras 180, 181
breasts 180–81
breathing 149, 188, 193
bride: budget bridal beauty 46–8
bronzers 28, 50, 52, 53, 58, 60, 130, 181
brushes: body 138; facial 75; hair 108,
    110, 111; lip 64; make-up 30, 31, 53;
    skin-stimulation 71
budget shopping 23–9

caffeine 37, 144, 193
calcium 16, 21, 22
calendula cream 154
calorie-burning 168
camomile 72
carotenoids 13
cash sales 219
celebrity secrets, cut-price 198–205
cellulite 37, 138, 139, 142, 154, 158, 208
ceramides 35
cheeks 56, 60–61, 175, 176–7
cherry gelatine 203
Chinese medical centres 154
cigarettes 130, 142
cinnamon 63
cleansers 25, 82, 84, 187, 208
cleansing 68–72, 82
cocoa butter 167, 200
cod liver oil 211
coenzyme Q1 38, 215
coffee 142, 144, 186, 200
cold sore 187–8
colds 154
collagen 13, 35, 38, 110, 145, 212, 215
colour stick, multipurpose 49
compacts 61
compresses 83, 84, 91, 201
concealer 28, 49, 53–6, 182, 185, 188
confidence 147–51
cortisol 146
cosmetic powder 29
cotton buds (swabs) 31, 63, 187, 204
crow's-feet 13, 68, 91
curling irons 107

dancing 168
dandruff 99, 100, 102
dehydration 144, 182, 183, 186
dental care 10
depilatory creams 125
detoxifying 142, 145, 164, 191, 193–5
diet 143, 145, 146, 149, 194
dihydroxyacetone 36
discounts 217, 218, 219
DIY 172
DNA 40
dog-walkers 169

elastin 35, 38
electrolysis 34, 126
enzymes 40, 194
Epsom salts 182
essential oils 97, 107, 153
evening primrose 212
exercise 168–73, 193; DVDs 34
exfoliation 12, 37, 40, 51, 73–6, 84, 86,
    118, 123, 124, 126, 127, 140, 141,
    205, 207, 208
eye cream 91, 185, 205
eye pencils 59, 67
eyebrows: shaping 9, 52, 65–7, 174;
    tinted 59
eyelashes: curlers 32, 59; false 60; tinted
    202
eyeliner 29, 59, 180, 184, 190
eyes: bloodshot 184, 186; bright 90;
    dark shadows under 144; droopy 175;
    irritated 89; make-up 58–60; 'panda
    eyes' 202; puffy 37, 52, 89, 90, 175,
    184, 185; smoky 28, 48; soother 83,
    90; sore 184; tired 90, 184; under-eye
    bags 56, 174; under-eye circles 17, 55,
    90, 142
eyeshadow 49, 52, 58, 61, 184

face creams 80, 82, 174
face lotion 205
face masks 71, 80, 84–7, 89
face massage 155, 159
face powder 56–8, 61, 177, 178, 182

face wipes 51, 59
facelift, faked 173–5
facial oil 79, 84
facial sauna 32
facials 161, 163; do-it-yourself 82–4
fibre 20
fine lines 19, 86
fish 13, 21, 22, 41, 143, 145
flat irons 107
flu busters 182–4
fluoride/fluorine 15, 130
foot care 12, 118, 119, 121, 158
foot spas 32
foundation 8, 29, 46, 49, 53–7, 176, 177,
    182, 183, 190
fragrances 132–7
free radicals 12, 13, 38, 145
freebies 217, 219–20
frown lines 173
fruit 13, 15, 16, 143, 144, 145, 191, 193;
    in face masks 84–7
fruit juice 194

garlic 15
glycerine 96, 123
grape-seed extract 215
gripper knickers 181
gyms 168, 172, 173

haggling 215, 217, 218, 219
hair: blow-drying 10, 33, 47, 111, 112,
    117, 149; bridal 46, 47; colour &
    highlights 104–7, 116, 117; conditioner
    21, 24, 96, 98, 99, 112, 123, 201; curls
    51, 108, 111, 112, 200; cuts 102–3,
    113–16, 176, 204; dry/greasy 24; fine
    52; fringe (bangs) 46, 102, 115; frizzy
    8, 51, 53, 108, 111; haircare 20–21;
    healthy 92–5; masks 99–102; oily 96,
    99; plaiting (braiding) 117; and prenatal
    vitamins 199; shiny 39, 107, 203; split
    ends 8, 11, 100, 101; strength 209;
    styling 107–12, 113, 178; tangles 110;
    value hair treatments 113–17; volume
    109, 208; waves 45, 201

hair bands 108, 117
hair gel 110
hair mousse 109, 111
hair-removal hints 123–7
hairdryers 33, 34, 107
hairspray 51, 107, 108, 109
hand blender 191
hand lotions 53, 120
hands, exfoliation of 118
hangover, hiding a 185–7
hats 8, 92
head massage 157
heel scrub 118
herbal mist 166
highlighters 49, 174, 177, 178
holistic therapist 152
housework 169
humectants 40
hyaluronic acid 38
hydration 10, 14, 17, 20, 29,
    37, 120

ice bath 186
iron 15, 17, 22

juicer 191
junk food 143

keratin 21, 110

labelling, lazy 216
laughter lines 175
lemon juice 52
lighting 146, 163
lip balm 11, 58, 64, 184, 201
lip brush 64
lip gloss 9, 28, 63, 179, 201
lip plumper 63
lip-fillers, fake 179–80
lipliners 63, 179
lips, super-soft 202
lipsticks 50, 59, 62–5, 130, 179, 184,
    188, 202
liver-cleansing 193
loyalty cards 163

lycopene 14
lymphatic drainage 138

magnesium 211
mailing lists 24, 163, 218
make-up: accentuate the positive 151;
    bridal 46, 47, 48; buying 27; make-up
    makeover 42–6; minimal 9, 194; no
    make-up 151; sleeping in 11; storage
    30; using differently 151
make-up bags 31
manicure 121, 122, 161
market research 220
mascara 9, 26, 48, 59, 60, 187, 190, 209
massage 33, 82, 119, 138, 155–61, 164
massage oil 157
melasma 146
milk 19, 198
milk of magnesia 70
mineral oil 39
minerals 19, 210
mirrors 33
moisturizers 11, 27, 28, 29, 53, 55, 71,
    76, 77–9, 87, 119, 142, 183, 185,
    190, 197
morning wake-up call 140
mouth spray 131
mouthwashes 129
muffin-top 181
muscular aches and pains 139

nail polish (varnish) 11, 28, 53, 59, 121,
    161
nails: biting 130; cuticles 119, 121; electric
    manicure 31; nail art 122; nail buffer 9;
    nailcare 21–3, 120–22, 198, 208, 211
nature 195
neutral colours 24
night cream 82
nose 177–8, 184
nuts 14, 17, 21, 41, 146

obesity 145
oil-free products 205
olive oil 203

omega-3s 13, 21, 41, 145, 211
omega-6s 41
online prices 217
oxygen 40, 82

packaging 28, 217
panthenol (vitamin B5) 39
pectin 132
pedicure 12, 46, 119, 122, 161
pedometer 34
peptides 40
perfumes 132–7
petroleum jelly 51, 58, 62, 63, 131, 137, 188, 204
phosphorus 22
polyphenols 15, 40
posture 8, 150, 181
probiotics 211
processed food 143, 193
promotions 24, 116, 220
protein 13, 21

quiffs 109

reader's trial panels 220
reflexology 153
resveratrol 13, 199
retinoids 35, 80
reward cards 24

sales 218
salt 175, 193, 194; 210
samples 24, 27, 46, 109, 217, 219, 220
scars 17, 19
scissors, hairstyling 33
scrubs 73–6, 118, 138, 139, 141, 166
seafood 19, 22
seaweed 167
selenium 14, 22, 212
serums 77, 78, 82, 84, 111
shampoo 25, 27, 52, 96, 97, 98, 105; dry 185, 190
shaving 123
shopping, budget 23–9
silica 20, 212

skin: dead skin cells 141; dry 15, 38, 56, 64, 70, 77, 119, 138, 140, 154, 166, 183, 186, 187; hydration 17, 37, 70, 145, 185; mature 56; oily 55, 70; pale 15, 17, 145, 182, 188, 201; purification 195; skincare 9, 17, 19, 146; sore 86, 89, 183; sunburnt 86, 89; supplements 210; tired 82, 85; toner 19, 55, 68, 70, 72, 84, 164
sleep 142, 193, 205; disguising a sleepless night 184–5
smiling 9, 151, 175
smoking 130, 142
soaps 69
spas 161, 162, 163–4, 166–7
special offers 27
SPF (sun protection factor) 11, 79, 92, 195, 196, 213
spider veins 13
sports goods 171
spots (pimples) 12, 17, 19, 51, 88–9, 110, 199
squats, shaping 182
stains 48
stairs 170, 171
steaming 83
stomach 181–2
straighteners, ceramic 35
straightening irons 51
stress 72, 146, 175
stretch marks 17, 140
sugar 145, 193
sugaring 125, 127
sulphur 22
sun damage 13, 17, 36
sun protection 195–7
sunglasses 91
sunscreen 11, 25, 37, 195–7
sweating 195

tanning, home 28, 31, 141, 142, 213
tea: for fragrant feet 118; green 15, 19, 139, 141, 193; herbal 90, 97, 164, 191, 195; mint 200; teabag toner 62
tea tree oil 51, 129, 205

teeth: care of 10, 15–16, 128–32; whitening treatments 128–31
threading 127
tired body 148
toenail fungus 119
tongue 195
toothbrushes 33, 75, 128, 129, 195
toothpaste 128, 129, 130, 198, 199
towels 163, 167
traditional Chinese medicine 156
trampoline 182
tummy tuck, faked 181–2
tweezers 35, 65, 67

ultraviolet (UV) rays 8, 91, 195
underwear 150

vegetable juice 191
vegetables 12–15, 19, 21, 143, 144, 193
vitamins 85, 199, 210; A (retinol) 22, 35, 121, 214; B group 17, 21, 22, 23, 214; B3 (niacin) 37; B5 (panthenol) 39; B6 99; B12 23; C 13, 17, 19, 38, 82, 194, 212; D 145; E 14, 17, 36, 73, 82, 99, 119, 200, 214; K 19
vouchers 220

water, drinking 10, 20, 164, 182, 186, 191, 201
waxing 124–7; eyebrow 67
weight loss 145
weight-training 170
wholegrains 143, 193
witch hazel 55, 123
wrinkles 9, 12–15, 19, 29, 68, 80, 142, 144, 145, 207, 212, 214

yoga 146

zinc 19, 21, 22, 212
zinc oxide 37